Go with the Flow

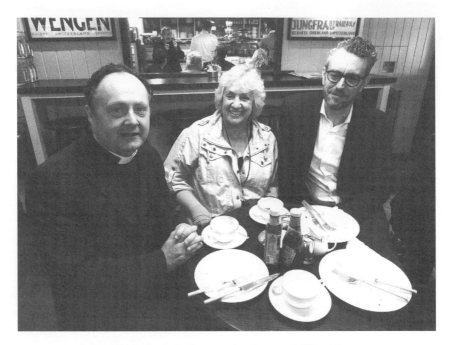

James Woodward, Gemma Levine and Clive Gregory
at the Mount Street Deli. Photographed by
Terry O'Neill who is reflected in the mirror

Go with the Flow

GEMMA LEVINE

QUARTET

The publication of this book has been
sponsored by Leaders in Oncology Care. All
royalties will be donated by the author to
Maggie's Cancer Caring Centres

First published in 2012 by
Quartet Books Limited
A member of the Namara Group
27 Goodge Street, London W1T 2LD

A catalogue record for this book
is available from the British Library

ISBN 978 0 7043 7260 3

Typeset by Antony Gray
Printed and bound in Great Britain by
T J International Ltd, Padstow, Cornwall

Contents

For my two sons, James and Adam Levine,
of whom I am so proud and to whom
I am so grateful for their care, encouragement,
support and sense of humour

Introduction

'You have cancer,' I was bluntly told: words that transform your world forever. Members of my family and some close friends are doctors and they would later confirm that it is not always easy to break the news with any less impact. Minimising or making light of this diagnosis can be patronising and disrespectful. One is left completely numb, dazed and shattered, and in my case, I gravitated to my bed and remained there for three entire days. I barely spoke to a soul, my appointments went unattended and my appetite had vanished.

I am a professional photographer and for over forty-five years have spent my life capturing images and exceptional moments. I specialised as a portrait photographer, having first commenced with three pictorial publications on the sculptor, Henry Moore.

I was married for twenty-five years and then divorced. I have two sons, James and Adam. James is a professor of endocrinology at the Mayo Clinic in the USA and Adam, a theatrical director living and based in Oslo, Norway. Both sons have been a complete inspiration and an unfailing support at every turn of events.

Diagnosed with cancer instantly forces you into a patient role, plunging you into a daunting, frightening and completely unknown new world. Life changes dramatically and suddenly you are faced with many unwelcome options and unlimited questions to be asked: What will the treatment involve? How does chemotherapy help and in what way? What is it like to undergo radiotherapy? How does it work? What are the side effects? Will I be able to tolerate the treatments? Will I have trained people to turn to and discuss things with at each stage? And, most of all, the fear of thinking – will I survive to be one of the lucky ones?

There is only one answer to that question . . . 'YES'.

The reason that this book is so important to me is that now I am more than a spectator and I can share the reality from the depths of my own experience. When people say to me, 'I know exactly what you are going through,' or, 'My friend has exactly the same cancer as you,' I am irritated and turn away. No two patients are ever the same and each person's experience is unique. Joanna Lumley so helpfully told me: 'The important thing is that people understand that it's a process that has to be gone through, not a ghastly battle that you win or lose.'

The Chief Rabbi, Lord Jonathan Sacks, told me he had cancer twice: 'I went with the flow which carried me through. I looked at the angel eyeball to eyeball, one of us blinked and it wasn't me . . . I refused.'

All my life I have worked on images and the power they create. It is said that a picture says more than a thousand words. The purpose of this book is to share my personal experience of breast cancer through the spectrum of photographs and try to alleviate the fear and void of the unknown.

Despite the initial shock and occasional overwhelming anxiety, I have grown and been transformed in many ways which I could never have imagined or expected. Above all, I have had some unique encounters, meeting many extraordinary people along the way who have enriched my life by their skills, integrity and devotion.

Following this Introduction, I write about my experience in two parts: one at the start and the second at the book's conclusion. The interim chapters are a potpourri of personal statements, with photographs, written by the experts. I encourage you to embrace the positive and dynamic achievements which medicine in this country, and in today's world, has to offer us.

All royalties and proceeds from this publication are donated to charity. I searched far and wide to find a charity to complement this book and to help those, like myself, guidng them through the stages of, and post, diagnosis, with care and expert knowledge, with the comfort of a unique homely environment. Maggie's Cancer Caring Centres, within the grounds of NHS hospitals, was the answer for me.

I finish by reiterating: we are all different and our journeys will carry us along different routes. Whoever you are, whatever your background and at whatever junction, we all basically have the same goal in mind: proceed, succeed and lead a full and normal life.

GEMMA LEVINE

Foreword: 1

DANIEL HOCHHAUSER

Cancer retains a fearsome reputation among diseases. The word itself, with its underlying connotations of insidiousness, pain and relentlessness, is responsible for this, together with a persistent notion that cancer treatments are frequently worse than the disease itself. Until relatively recently this resulted in a lack of open discussion with patients diagnosed with cancer. When I was a medical student in the 1980s it was common to euphemistically refer to patients on ward rounds as having been diagnosed with a 'mitotic lesion' (mitosis being the process by which cells divide), rather than to mention cancer. This reticence has essentially gone over the past

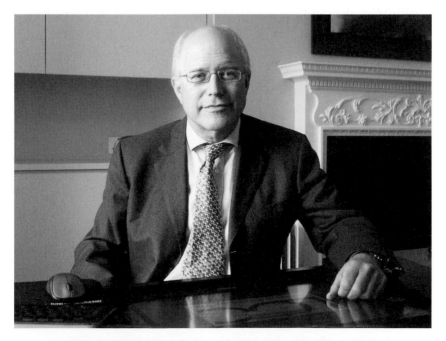

PROFESSOR DANIEL HOCHHAUSER DPhil, FRCP
*Kathleen Ferrier Professor of Medical Oncology and Consultant
Medical Oncologist, UCL Cancer Institute and UCLH Trust*

decades and it is now universally recognised that frank and honest discussion of diagnosis, treatment and prognosis (when requested) is essential.

Increased awareness of cancer has arisen as a result of several processes. A critical factor has undoubtedly been the publication of many autobiographical accounts of encounters with cancer, best exemplified by John Diamond's powerful memoir of his illness. These *pathographies* have resulted in a more widespread understanding of cancer, not least in underlining the role of the patient in making decisions on treatment. The role of friends, family and the critical effects on emotional and psychological wellbeing on cancer patients are now also apparent. Additionally there is an increased awareness by patients of the implications of diagnosis and generally a more questioning attitude towards treatment options.

Gemma Levine is an outstanding photographer with an international reputation. Her subjects range from Henry Moore and through three decades of portraits of famous people to contemporary images of Israel, and are always marked by her own personal imaginative flair and creativity. When Gemma was diagnosed with breast cancer, as she vividly recalls, the process of becoming a cancer patient involved entry into a 'completely unknown new world'. When the initial trauma passed, she saw this as an opportunity to focus on producing a collection of images and essays which would provide a sense of the full range of experiences during her treatment for cancer. Gemma has brought together the team involved in her care to cover key aspects of the subject to produce this personal perspective, including aspects of care which are generally unappreciated. This allows the subject material to encompass basic medical and surgical issues together with spiritual and psychological aspects. What is unusual is the inclusion of sections on practical ways to enhance a patient's quality of life, ranging from swimwear through podiatry and scalp cooling. The pervasive attitude of Gemma's approach is an essential optimism illustrated by her title *Go with the Flow*. Visual images, as always in Gemma's work, provide the unifying central feature through which the cancer experience is understood. This ranges from lesser known subjects such as the development of cooling caps for patients receiving chemotherapy, through to what we now recognise as being crucial, the physical surroundings in which cancer care is provided. A clean, modern and well-designed environment provides the necessary location where care is provided. Treatment of cancer is rarely a single event in which a treatment is provided and the patient discharged. In reality the cancer experience, or 'journey' as it is often known, consists of a number of interactions with different professionals at different times but within a single location. The experience of a cancer patient does not end with the cessation of treatment. Transition to 'wellness' often requires help in allowing the individual to return to normal life without the constant monitoring and clinic visits which occur while treatment is in progress.

The contributors to this volume write on subjects that were significant in Gemma's own experience of breast cancer. However, at the centre of the book is the scientific medical foundation which made possible the progress made in the management of patients with cancer. The key to the dramatic changes in the management of cancer over the past decades has undoubtedly been the increased scientific understanding of how cancers develop. Our ability to understand the alterations in DNA, the genetic material found in all cells, which result in cancers has been fundamental in allowing us both to understand how cancers develop and to devise novel treatments. Without such understanding it would not be possible to move forward with radical changes to the ways in which cancers are diagnosed and treated. Many of the initially effective treatments for cancer were obtained serendipitously and resulted in chemo-therapy drugs which proved dramatically effective in several cancers such as testicular cancer and Hodgkin's disease. The development and testing of chemotherapeutic agents during the 1970s and '80s resulted in good responses to treatment for several cancers but chemotherapy alone was unable to cure patients with more advanced disease.

Despite the great advances in laboratory research, the foundation of effective treatment for most cancers, including breast cancer, remains surgery. Although for over a century this has been recognised as the only way to achieve cure of breast cancers, it is only in the past several decades, with the results of large clinical trials, that it has become recognised that less extensive procedures can be performed.

The introduction of lumpectomy and the reduced extent of mastectomies, with the abandoning of the radical operations previously performed, has had a dramatic impact on quality of life for millions of women. Surgical innovation continues with research indicating that less lymph nodes require removal in many cases, as well as the challenging surgery of breast reconstruction which has further improved quality of life for patients with breast cancer.

Although surgery remains the only way to cure breast cancer, it is clear that in a number of patients there is a significant risk of the cancer returning despite apparently successful surgery. The introduction of large-scale studies in breast cancer patients has conclusively demonstrated the benefits of both hormonal and chemotherapy treatments in preventing recurrence of cancer. This has allowed intelligent risk-stratified use of chemotherapy. Patients who are defined as having a higher risk of the cancer recurring are offered chemotherapy to reduce the probability of this happening. Despite this important advice it has become clear that chemotherapy has limitations apart from the often serious side effects associated with treatment. Some patients receive treatment which may not have been necessary, because the tests available to identify patients at higher risk are not accurate enough. Hence the major efforts in developing 'biomarkers', a simple test of the tumour, looking at the genetic alterations of the cancer to provide a clue as to whether the cancer will behave more or less aggressively.

Chemotherapy remains an important part of the treatment of breast cancer both in preventing recurrence and in the management of patients whose cancers have spread elsewhere. The main focus of current research and treatment, especially in breast cancer, is in the development of a personalised medicine approach. Rather than regarding all breast cancers as being the same, we are now able to define patients with different subgroups of cancers which will respond to specific therapies apart from chemotherapies. The best-known example, discovered several decades ago, was the under-standing of the importance of whether breast cancers expressed the oestrogen receptor which rendered them more sensitive to treat-ment with agents such as Tamoxifen. Another critical discovery was that the antibody Herceptin (trastuzumab) could be effective for patients whose cancers express a specific protein (HER2) which is targeted by the drug. These two findings alone have revolutionised treatment for women with breast cancer, and the aim of the coming years is to investigate whether there are other specific alterations in breast cancers which can be targeted by the many new agents now being tested.

Thus far, I have focused on the critical role of scientific research and development in improving diagnosis and treatment of cancer. Only rigorous research will allow the development of new therapies, and only well-conducted trials of these agents, to ensure that the right patients receive the right treatments thereby avoiding both ineffective and needlessly toxic treatments of those who would not benefit. Additionally we have a responsibility to carefully monitor the expense and cost to society of these new agents before they are introduced into the clinic.

However, it is clear that whilst scientific and medical advances are the key foundations for treatment of cancer, there are many other crucial factors to consider. The treatment plan of the cancer patient involves a team of professionals with disparate but complementary skills to optimise quality of life. The administration of chemotherapy is a complex and highly skilled process requiring not only a deep understanding of the technical aspects but also the management of both common and rare side effects. That is why the chemotherapy nurse specialist plays such a vital role in care of patients. It is obvious that these skills need to be combined with an empathic personality and the ability to communicate clearly and efficiently. Synergy between clinicians and nurse specialists is crucial in facilitating the optimal management of the illness. The presence of a multidisciplinary team is an absolute necessity for the provision of efficient and humane cancer care.

There are several other aspects for the optimisation of care of breast cancer patients. From the time of diagnosis onwards, the psychological and emotional effects on individuals are profound. Many patients deal with these issues themselves and rely additionally on the support of close family and friends. There are, however, a significant number of patients for whom expert advice is required. Psychological reactions are clearly altered by cultural and religious factors. This is why the emergent branch of psycho-oncology is of such importance in ensuring that the specific needs of cancer patients are met. With breast surgery and chemotherapy there are physical and psychological changes which directly affect sexuality, social interactions and family relationships. Additionally, differing religious perspectives provide multiple ways in which patients cope with diagnosis and treatment. For some the diagnosis of cancer reaffirms religious faith which provides a mode of belief through which the experience can be understood and accepted. For others there may be a resultant crisis of religious faith and the consequent distress may be difficult to deal with at the same time as often debilitating treatment.

It is the originality and imagination of Gemma Levine that has motivated her to provide such an unusual and humane overview of what breast cancer means to her, but which will undoubtedly be of great value to others touched by the disease. Above all she seeks to give a perspective whose aim is the healing of patients and to allow each patient the opportunity to move away from a purely passive acceptance of being a cancer patient into active involvement in management of their disease and to return to wellness as much as is feasible.

Acknowledgements

To friends who took an interest
over and above the call of duty:

Michael Bernstein, Rebecca Barrett, Terry Blatten,
Fridette Cain, Samantha Cameron,
Ali Cibich, Joseph Coté, Councillor Robert Davis,
Professor Paul Ellis, Ian Evans, Alex Ezeoke, Dave Foster,
Edward Friend, Sally Friend, Suzanne and Simon Friend,
Terry Hack, Gill Heighway, Nigel Hammond and team at
35 Grosvenor Square, Mary Hawtins, Lilian Hochhauser,
Jeremy King, Angela and Chris Knowles, Prue Leith,
Eric Levine, Maureen McGoldrick, Bernie Martin,
Dr Jonathan Moore, Dr S. Nazeer, Peter Osborne,
Vergie Palma, Madhu Parmar, Rachel Paul, Zelda Pomson,
Ros Roberts, Amanda Rose, Mike Shaw, Reg Shaw,
Denise Sinclair, Sir Harry Solomon,
Danielle Thompson, Nicki Thompson.

Chemo-Buddies – Friends who found the time
to sit with me during my chemotherapy
sessions at the LOC, London:

Barbara Cantello, James Levine, Lilian Hochhauser,
Mary Hawtins, Patricia Counsell, Sally Friend,
Sonia Shalam, Suzanne Friend, Zelda Pomson.

Sincere gratitude to some of my distinguished
sitters from my past publications, who have come
forward so enthusiastically to write the quotes which
head the chapters for this book:

Lady Mary Archer, Dame Joan Bakewell,
Baroness Betty Boothroyd, Simon Callow,
Helena Bonham Carter, Dame Judi Dench,

The Rt Hon. William Hague MP, Professor Lord Harries,
Gloria Hunniford, Boris Johnson, Dame Kiri Te Kanawa,
Felicity Kendal, Baroness Glenys Kinnock, Prue Leith,
Joanna Lumley, The Rt Hon. Sir John Major, Terry O'Neill,
Sir Cliff Richard, Angela Rippon, Sir Richard Rogers,
The Chief Rabbi, Lord Jonathan Sacks, Jon Snow,
David Suchet, Kirsty Wark.

The publication of this book has been sponsored by
Leaders in Oncology Care. All proceeds and royalties
arising from the publication have been donated by
Gemma Levine to Maggie's Cancer Caring Centres.

I wish to thank BUPA for undertaking an active
interest in this enterprise.
'BUPA is committed to providing the best care available and is
proud to support Gemma Levine's *Go with the Flow*.'

And finally, with thanks to my publisher Naim Attallah
without whom this book would not exist.

Working with Maggie's Cancer Caring Centre, I want to acknowledge the thoughtfulness and expertise of their CEO, Laura Lee, and her associates, Georgina Annan, Katie Tait and Pam Richardson.

Having completed this book on 3 October 2011, I met quite incidentally a stranger and I think this short encounter will say more than any words I could describe.

At the NHS doctor's surgery I noticed a woman in a pink sweater, waiting as I was, to see the doctor. An hour later, walking home through Grosvenor Square, I realised I was just a footstep away from the lady in the pink sweater. I approached her and said, 'Haven't I just seen you at the surgery?'

'Yes,' she replied. I began to make light conversation about the weather as we were walking, and suddenly she turned to face me and said bluntly, 'I have cancer.'

I took a deep breath and took a long look at her. She appeared sad and drawn. I told her I was so sorry. She said she had little hope. I asked her if she had had any treatment? She said that the chemotherapy had reduced the tumour in her stomach.

After a long pause, I said to her: 'You must try to think positively.'

She said she had seen so many doctors and psychiatrists, but the only glimmer of light was that she had found, over the past few months, Maggie's Cancer Caring Centre in the grounds of the Charing Cross Hospital.

'Have you heard of it?' she asked. 'It has given me so much comfort and help.'

'Wow!' I said. Then I told her about this book and my experience.

Thank you, Angelina!

Foreword: 2

As architects, we aim to design healthcare facilities that offer both a sense of care and control for patients and meet the needs of the science of medicine. With the design of Maggie's London, we have sought to create a calm and welcoming home where those affected by cancer – as well as their families and friends – can meet and talk.

BARON ROGERS OF RIVERSIDE

Gemma's dynamic, creative and passionate character just burst out of her. She has found an inspiring new way of living with the consequences that a cancer diagnosis brings and is helping others by sharing her ideas with us in this great book. Her defiant determination to use her experience of cancer as a positive catalyst is both remarkable and noble and I encourage you to take the time to enjoy and savour what she shares with us in the following pages.

In *Go with the Flow* Gemma looks at all aspects of living with cancer – the emotional, psychological and practical. This is crucial because visitors to Maggie's network of Cancer Caring Centres tell me that facing all aspects of their lives, and having guidance to do so, is of fundamental value to them. As people rebuild their lives they often look to find a 'new normal' in the face of the uncertainty that cancer diagnosis and treatment have brought.

I started life as an oncology nurse and one of my most inspiring patients was Maggie Keswick Jencks. Working alongside her as we travelled to the United States and created a blueprint for a centre that would support patients to get the comprehensive care they needed to complement their NHS treatment was a privilege. As Maggie and the patients that followed her became active participants in their own treatment, there was a major turning point for people affected by cancer.

As the numbers of people diagnosed with cancer is growing so too are the numbers who are living with the disease. This means the significance of Maggie's work will only increase with time as the psychological and emotional support they need in order to maintain that all-important 'joy of living' is upheld and nurtured within the four walls of a Maggie's Centre.

But we can only grow thanks to generous supporters, like Gemma, who make Maggie's their beneficiary. Visitors to Maggie's and people affected by cancer will find great balm and hope through these pages. We are grateful to Gemma for her kind support and generosity and for creating an enjoyable and helpful tool for people living with cancer today.

LAURA LEE
CEO Maggie's Cancer Caring Centres

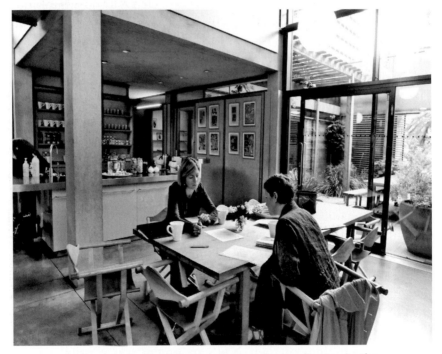

Laura Lee in the Maggie's Cancer Caring Centre in the grounds of the Charing Cross Hospital

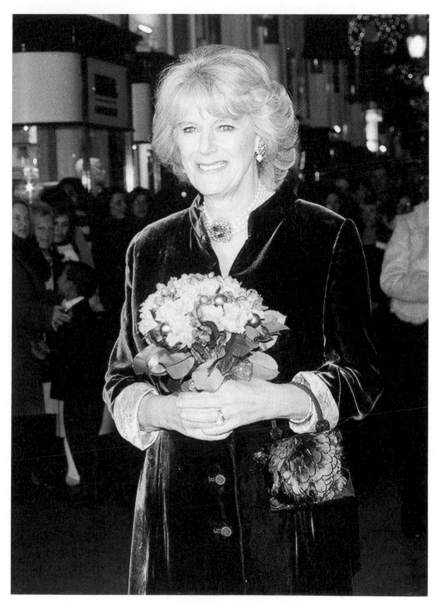

HRH THE DUCHESS OF CORNWALL
President of the Maggie's Cancer Caring Centres

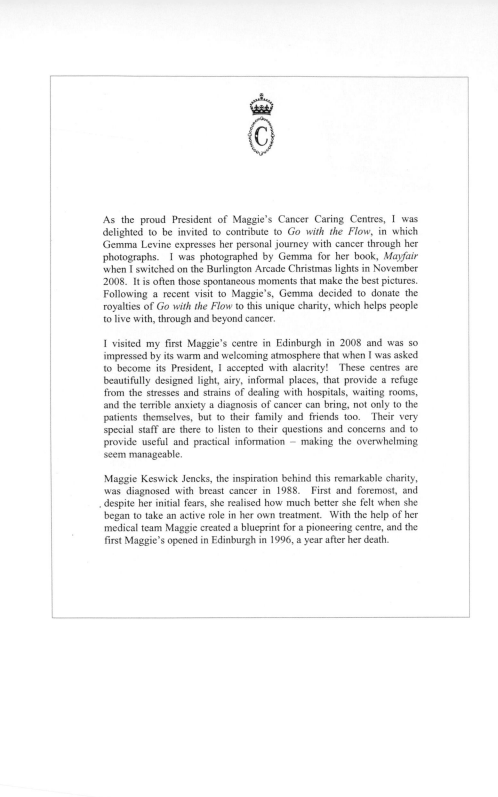

As the proud President of Maggie's Cancer Caring Centres, I was delighted to be invited to contribute to *Go with the Flow*, in which Gemma Levine expresses her personal journey with cancer through her photographs. I was photographed by Gemma for her book, *Mayfair* when I switched on the Burlington Arcade Christmas lights in November 2008. It is often those spontaneous moments that make the best pictures. Following a recent visit to Maggie's, Gemma decided to donate the royalties of *Go with the Flow* to this unique charity, which helps people to live with, through and beyond cancer.

I visited my first Maggie's centre in Edinburgh in 2008 and was so impressed by its warm and welcoming atmosphere that when I was asked to become its President, I accepted with alacrity! These centres are beautifully designed light, airy, informal places, that provide a refuge from the stresses and strains of dealing with hospitals, waiting rooms, and the terrible anxiety a diagnosis of cancer can bring, not only to the patients themselves, but to their family and friends too. Their very special staff are there to listen to their questions and concerns and to provide useful and practical information – making the overwhelming seem manageable.

Maggie Keswick Jencks, the inspiration behind this remarkable charity, was diagnosed with breast cancer in 1988. First and foremost, and despite her initial fears, she realised how much better she felt when she began to take an active role in her own treatment. With the help of her medical team Maggie created a blueprint for a pioneering centre, and the first Maggie's opened in Edinburgh in 1996, a year after her death.

The essence of *Go with the Flow* reflects the attitude held by Maggie Keswick Jencks, that "above all what matters is not to lose the joy of living in the fear of dying". A diagnosis of cancer can be frightening, but it is amazing how resilient people can be. I am touched by the courage, hope and determination which I have seen in the people who use the Maggie's centres and which continues to inspire me to support Maggie's. Gemma encapsulates this *joie de vivre* herself and articulates it so beautifully in this book.

Camilla

Breast Cancer – A Journey: Part One

GEMMA LEVINE

Illness is one of life's greatest trials, but friendship and family are rich consolations that make it possible to endure it with hope and dignity and to emerge from the other side.

THE RT HON. WILLIAM HAGUE MP FRSL

July–September 2010

Having been swimming in the early morning I discovered that one of my breasts was inflamed with defined red rims, much larger than the other and heavier in weight. Thinking I might have an infection my friend suggested I called my local NHS GP, Dr Nazeer. After an immediate brief exchange of words, I was told to visit him in his surgery at 8.30 am the next morning.

Dr Nazeer examined me and within an hour I was sitting nervously waiting to see a cancer specialist, Professor Mokbel, at the Princess Grace Hospital. I was scrutinised, probed, scanned, had biopsies taken. CT – MRI – PET scans. These abbreviated names, at the time, meant nothing to me. I was bluntly told, 'You have cancer.' Then, I was ushered into various consulting rooms and, within three hours, had several in-depth tests. The diagnosis was so formidable . . . so severe . . . so conclusive.

My long-standing and closest friend, Zelda, waited for me through-out and then drove me home. I went to bed, numb and in a complete daze. I could not reach my son James, as he was travelling, but I did reach Adam, my younger son, who took a flight from Oslo instantly to be with me at this terrifying time.

I do not remember those out-of-focus hours to this day, alerting me to the 'wake-up call' of my life. Certain things often change us radically and stay with us forever. We can never shut the door to life's complexities and horrors which are sure to haunt us in the days that follow. But I will certainly try to come to terms with all that has happened and what has reshaped my life so abruptly.

The following week my tests confirmed that I did in fact have breast cancer. I was sent to meet Professor Ellis at the London Oncology Clinic (LOC) in Harley Street. I took my sister, Sally, and her daughter-in-law, Suzanne, for support. The professor managed momentarily to relax me and explained in simple terms how he saw the progression of treatments at the Clinic, starting with chemotherapy once a week for twelve sessions, four hours at a time. This fearsome thought stayed with me continuously and I found the entirety of it unimaginable.

James, my son, a professor at the Mayo Clinic, arrived from the USA and together we entered the LOC to meet Michael Jones, RGN, who explained the procedure and answered any questions as we talked. It was very helpful James being there as he was able to fully concentrate. I was not. Sinister thoughts, darting to and fro, anxiously remained with me until I embarked on the first seven-hour session of chemotherapy a week later. In fear of the unknown, during those foremost anxious hours, I was immensely grateful for my son being at my side.

Life changed dramatically. It was an unconditional surrender. I began to reflect on the purpose and richness of my life, all the passions and aspirations, all the setbacks, the love that came and went. I started to evaluate relationships – family who had been a witness to my life and mine to theirs.

First and foremost my two sons, who had always been an inspiration as far as I was concerned, were now to become an inspiration to those who surrounded me. The elder, James, lives in the USA and the younger, Adam, in Norway. Both have full lives with fulfilling jobs. They have constantly caught flights to be with me. Not easy for them, but a tower of strength for me. The warmth and caring they have shown have been a major influence in helping me to deal with this frightening situation.

I quickly discovered who my genuine friends were. Dedication, warmth, and an unequivocal sensitivity had seeped through. The one element I could not, and will not, endure is negativity. I am striving with all my strength to be positive and therefore cannot tolerate being dragged down by gloomy counterproductive weakness. Therefore a few – a very few – have fallen from their heights and out of my life. Inevitably, I leant on the shoulder of my local GP,

Dr Nazeer. Without doubt he played a leading part. He was constantly at the end of the telephone night and day to talk and to calm me. His concern and positive common sense lifted a great weight off my mind. He met my sons and formed friendships with both of them.

*   *   *

My first experience prior to the treatment was being sent to the Cromwell Hospital to have a *portacath* fitted. It is a soft plastic tube tunnelled under the skin of the chest. The tip of the catheter lies in a large vein just above the heart and the other end connects with the *port*. It is used to give the chemotherapy treatment, an easier way than to put needles frequently into veins in the arms. Professor Ellis suggested that this was a good thing. I was apprehensive of the unknown. In order gently to persuade me he assured me that I would like this particular doctor, as he was 'good looking and all the women patients flocked to him'. There had to be some incentive for me to go through this!

Having become reconciled to the initial trauma and the knowledge I was a victim of this terrible disease, I have learnt to live with the day-by-day routine of the changes to my life. What do I fear the most? I guess it is the natural thought that maybe I won't be one of the lucky ones. But now, today, I am over half way through my chemotherapy and feel positive, content and fully aware of the changes to my body and my life. I was mortified to learn that my hair would thin and drop out. It would have a huge effect on my self-confidence, above everything. I shuddered at the thought of buying a wig or walking around with a head totally bare.

I discovered that the clinic could provide me with a helmet, which they call a *cold cap*. This looks like a racing bike helmet, weighing almost a kilo. It is placed firmly on the head and strapped under the chin. When in position, the temperature inside the cap drops to 8 degrees below zero, cold and onerous. The cap was unbearable to start with but soon became acceptable. I thought if this would prevent my hair falling out, to endure the discomfort for three hours once a week, it would have to be.

There are many rules for hair care in this situation. No use of a hair dryer, no styling with a brush, no colouring, no chemicals, no

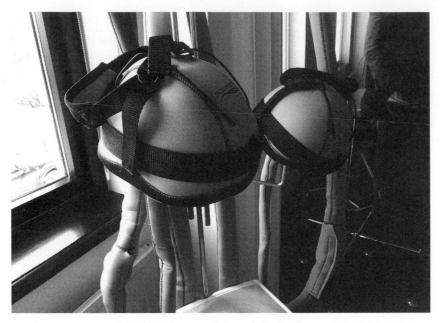

Paxman – cold cap helmets

pulling or tugging. I was told to use simple shampoos and no other products. I simply wash my hair each day, towel dry and scrunch it. During the hours of wearing the cold cap, I am wrapped up in blankets and given hand warmers. I am served the most delicious hot chocolate and told to 'hold the thought' of the sun setting across the lagoon towards the Basilica Della Salute, where Monet had a studio and painted the exquisite variegated shades of the whimsical sunset across the lagoon in Venice. That recollection of moments I had experienced each year for forty years carried me through the brutal reality. It is a severe process which I am forced to endure at this time.

A nutritionist came to visit me and told me of the few food items I could not eat and the vast amount of foods that were acceptable. All my life, periodically, I had been watching a diet and now for the first time in years I had been let loose to enjoy such things as cake, chocolates, bread, potatoes, baked beans . . . all the foods I love, so this was a major plus. Another large plus was that I could drink champagne and wine (but in moderation, of course!).

The Oncology Clinic, each week, provided me with medication for any of the foreseeable medical problems that might arise.

Having the right medication at hand would prevent me from worrying about where to find the right antibiotic, for example in the middle of the night or if I was marooned on a desert island! Going away for a weekend break, I needed a separate travel bag to accommodate all the medication. The tablet I like the most is an anti-sickness pill called *Dom Pérignon* . . . Oh, no, mistake. It's called *Domperidone*!

The significant change for me is fatigue. I tire more easily and have regular afternoon bedrest and early nights. I was told by Dr Alison, at the LOC, that 'The nap is the key.' I do rise early each morning to swim at 6 am. Swimming is idyllic for me. I swim for twenty minutes and then exercise for twenty minutes.

In my 30s, I used to go to a Swedish exercise class called *Mensendick* – the discipline which I have now readapted into a simple pool application and I do this regularly each day. (This is equally efficient out of water.) I have found, in my present situation, that this helps me enormously to relax, hence my movements are not as stiff as they might be otherwise. At the end of the book, I have noted down the exercises. I would suggest this to anyone as I am sure it has made an enormous difference to my wellbeing and my day.

Mentally, I am less tolerant. I cannot wait in queues, or on-line. I cannot dial numbers that put you through umpteen different options, so I simply press O for a voice and if I don't succeed, I hang up. I cannot wait for eggs to boil for four minutes, so I eat them after three. I used to love burnt toast, now I eat toast as soft bread.

When people say: 'I hope you don't mind me telling you, but my friend has exactly the same cancer as you . . . ' I turn away and become agitated. Or, 'I know exactly how you feel.' That is another major irritation. I am fearful to read newspapers. An article on cancer makes me nervous. It seems every day the newspaper reporters are giving cancer patients something 'to do or not to do', 'to eat or not to eat'!

No two patients are the same, or have the same degree of illness, or have the same treatment or cocktail of medication. All our treatments are varied according to our, age, health, weight and so on. We are all different. My friend, Paulette Baukol of the Mayo Clinic cancer division, says: 'We know quite a bit about how to prevent certain cancers but we often don't know how to "individualise" the message or the specific dose of preventive medicine or how to tailor that prevention, even though the saying is "an ounce of prevention . . . " to prevent cancers we do not even know about.'

For so many, as with me, living alone is a major problem. During the day I am strong. The nights are completely different. For moments fear and panic grip me, coupled with sinister thoughts. The disadvantage of not having a partner is apparent. There is no one to share.

I cannot endure sleeping pills and they do not agree with me. I have compromised on an herbal pill called *Valerian*. It does relax me but does not help maintain a full six hours' sleep. I awake on two or three occasions in the night, toss and turn, make tea and usually watch a *Columbo* on TV. Nights are difficult. I feel powerless in my dreams and wait for dawn to break.

My days are fully occupied as I make sure I have plenty to do. At first, when I met with Professor Ellis and learnt a little of the forthcoming events for me, I remember saying to him that I wanted to live my life as normally as possible, being as active, physically and mentally, as I was before. I realise now that this is not feasible.

I do not have the strength or stamina to work in my field as a photographer. Two weeks into chemotherapy, an American girl friend burst insensitively into my flat. 'I must have some photographs taken right now! I need a glamorous session for a magazine.' My spirits fell as I realised that I lacked energy, even to lift my Hasselblad from its case. I said to her, 'I can hardly boil an egg, let alone undertake a photo shoot.'

Mentally, I am able to adapt my thoughts regarding office matters which need daily attention. Working on the computer does not tire me. I do not like talking on the telephone. I cannot pass the time of day with idle gossip and what I find totally impossible is responding to an argument. I simply can't participate. I feel fragile, my throat tightens and I fade.

What I am about to say now might sound very strange. But instead of dreading each Tuesday, which is my 'Chemo Day', I somewhat look forward to it. Each week I had asked a different friend to sit with me for an hour (Chemo Buddies). I look forward to varied conversations as my friends hold different jobs and different

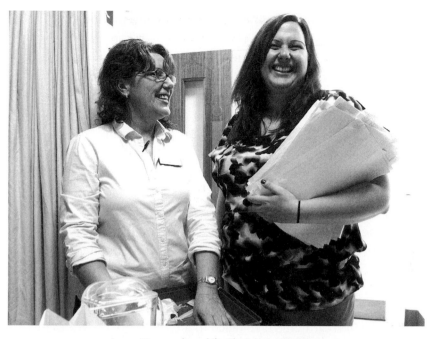

Jane Kennedy with Christina de Silva

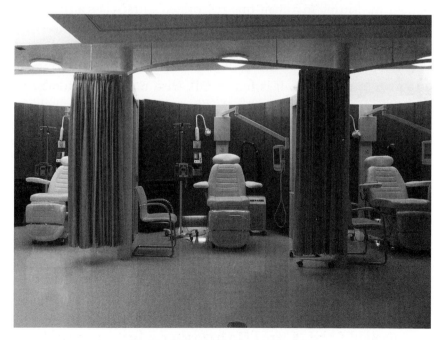

Chemotherapy chairs at the LOC

professions and I enjoy hearing their stories and momentarily being thrust into their worlds.

I have asked some of my friends to tell me how they feel about visiting me in treatment. Mary said she was saddened by the fact that each cubicle was occupied. It was like a 'fully packed auditorium,' Sonia said. 'Stepping into a space filled with patients all undergoing chemotherapy was daunting – a certain quietness prevailed in the whole ward, a veil had been lifted from over me. I had stepped into the unknown to make my way to Gemma's side, leaving my fears behind.'

Suzanne said she thought she would be frightened to see my appearance in my '8 degrees below freezing' cap. But pleasantly surprised to see me, she wrote: 'In her discreet cubicle – looking just like Gemma, but with a red-looking swimming cap covering her head, strapped lightly round the chin. It was certainly not a sight to be shocked by; in fact I thought she looked rather cute!'

The actual treatments take place in a basement, a sparkling white setting with bright light coming through skylights overhead. Each patient was sitting in a chair that resembled a first-class airline seat. There is a buzz of activity, not noisy, but congenial. Staff are serving drinks to patients and guests and chatting as if old friends.

The nursing staff at the LOC could not be more caring or attentive to my needs. It is fun to talk with my weekly nurse and look forward to chatting with her. The nurses are thorough. They explain about the drugs they administer and point out the side effects. I am at ease talking to them and do not feel inhibited asking questions. However busy they are, they always seem to have time to explain. The 'team', as they call themselves, is headed by Michael Jones, who is positive and such an enthusiast.

I realise how fortunate I am that I have subscribed to BUPA health insurance. Without years of annual regular payments I could not have been able to afford such 'luxury' care at this time. I am so grateful for this privilege. It seemed all my adult life I had subscribed to private medicine but also, on a regular basis, I have used the NHS. At a moment's notice, I can take a five-minute walk to my local medical centre, where I can have regular health tests or checks and feel comforted by the fact that they are instantly there for me.

*   *   *

I had often wondered about cancer patients who needed chemotherapy and lived in areas that were vast distances from hospitals. I discovered quite by chance, by reading the New Year's Honours list that a lady Christine Mills MBE had lost her husband to cancer and one of the many stresses was travelling sixty miles from their home to their nearest oncology centre.

Mrs Mills was inspired by a vision, by Dr Sean Elyan, to bring chemotherapy closer to the patient. She launched in 2007 the first mobile chemotherapy unit and formed a charity 'Hope for Tomorrow'.

The units are operated by highly trained NHS staff, and they can travel five days a week throughout their counties of operation to five set locations. These units have the capacity to treat up to twenty patients a day.

I feel this operation is one of the most rewarding and positive modern achievements. So many thanks to Christine Mills the founder and her Chairman Lord MacLaurin.

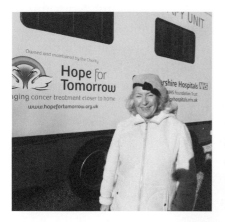 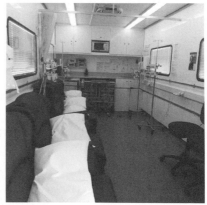

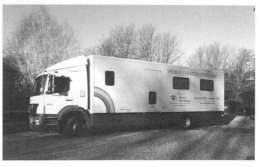

Above: Christine Mills *right*: the 'Hope for Tomorrow' mobile unit and, *above right;* its interior

*   *   *

Now that the final twelfth chemotherapy approaches, I am naturally becoming very nervous of the prognosis. During the treatment I lulled myself into a state of acceptance. Has the chemo worked? I feel so good. Is this a positive – or a negative? Of course there have been times when I have been near to tears. I have turned the telephone off as I cannot bear to hear myself repeat constantly the state of my health. I become demoralised and close to an anxiety attack.

My son James pointed out to me that during this period, from the time I was diagnosed until now, our roles have been reversed. He explained, kindly, that in his eyes I had become the child and he the parent. I know he was right; even though there is no need at this time for explanation, one's sense of self changes and one cannot help being excessively nervous of the unknown. Tragedy we can choose to be bewildered by or we just carry on and hopefully, with courage and strength, look forward to sunnier days.

Today, with only one week left of chemotherapy treatment, I spent the day in the country at Bliss Mill, Chipping Norton (see pp 182–3), sitting in the late afternoon sun, under a swaying willow tree, watching the ducks gliding through the water lilies along the length of the pond, towards their nest in the bulrushes. It was serene and peaceful and I can only long for the time when I can revisit this idyllic setting without apprehension.

A Patient's Journey

MIKE JONES RGN
Oncology Care in Harley Street

We are living in a time of amazing breakthroughs in the care of control of cancer. Let us be grateful to be here today and support as much as we can the research and work that will allow even more of us to survive tomorrow.

FELICITY KENDAL CBE

Hello, my name is Mike Jones; I am the Deputy Head of Clinical Services and nurse team leader at Leaders in Oncology Care in Harley Street. I joined the team nearly six years ago, shortly after the clinic opened in May 2005. My background is almost exclusively working in cancer / HIV care since qualifying as a nurse in 1993.

I have worked in many capacities in most of the major London hospitals over the last eighteen years and feel myself very fortunate to be working for an organisation which prides itself on providing quality care for patients receiving treatment for cancer. I work as part of a team of people who all play a part in making LOC the success it is.

Our vision and philosophy of care are based on providing excellence in care quality for the patient and their individual needs. The people who attend LOC all have very differing and individual needs as we treat people at very different stages of their disease and treatment. We often invite patients before they start treatment to visit the clinic and meet the team and it was in this capacity that I first had the pleasure of meeting Gemma and her son for a pre-chemo assessment.

The First Visit

Meeting patients, families and friends before treatment begins is an important introduction to the planned treatment and the

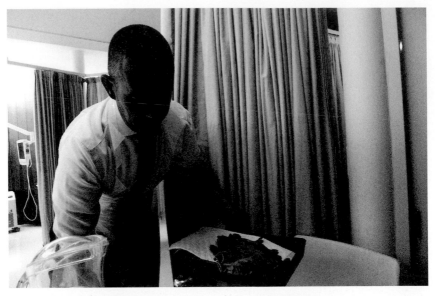

Mike Jones in attendance at treatment

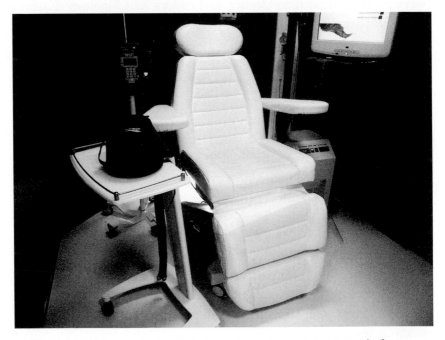

My chemotherapy chair at the LOC. With the cold cap ready for use

environment and support where the care will be delivered. It is often a very anxious and distressing time for patients who may have had very little time since diagnosis of their cancer to deal with all the information and proposed treatment that is being offered. This is an opportunity based on the individual patient's needs to help answer questions, address fears and concerns, and discuss potential side effects and the management of common symptoms. It is an opportunity to advise and inform the patient on their treatment plan and identify the role that the LOC team will have in their care.

In helping to explain the role of chemotherapy it is often helpful to give a brief explanation of the principles of treatment, with a basic discussion on the biology of cancer.

Cell Biology

Cancer is a disease which originates in the cell and the mechanism in which the cell divides. Cells are very small, very specialised and vast in numbers. As a normal state of growth and repair they have a lifespan. Cancer, in its very simple definition, is where for whatever reason this normal cell cycle is disrupted and the cell exceeds its normal lifespan and continues to divide and replicate. This continued growth and division after a time can cause clumps of abnormal cells to form a mass, or tumour, which can continue to grow. The human body has many types of cells, each specialised to its function, for example liver, brain, muscle and bone. All types of cells rely on the process of cell division to replace damaged and old cells, and therefore all have the potential for these cells to have this process disrupted, altered and to become cancerous.

Even at a stage where these cancerous cells have become tumours, they are so small they are unnoticed and asymptomatic. It is often only when these tumours have grown large enough to notice, that is, lumps or bumps, or are having an impact on other organs causing symptoms, that investigations begin. It should be mentioned that not all cancers form tumours, and that some cancer is a malignancy of the blood or lymph system. We treat both forms of cancer, that is, solid tumours, such as breast, lung, ovary, prostate and colon/upper GI; or haematology disorders such as leukaemias and lymphomas.

Cancer treatment is very individual to the patient. It relies on many different factors, that is, the type of cancer, location, size, or involvement of other organs. It also relies on the individual and their current health status and their individual preferences. Cancer treatment often involves different specialists working in collaboration (multi-disciplinary teams) providing part of the treatment plan for the management of the cancer. The specialities include investigations / staging, surgery, radiotherapy and chemotherapy.

Investigations / Disease Staging

The scrutiny of the patient's individual disease / tumour, often through a minor procedure such as a biopsy either of the primary tumour or associated lymph glands, will give important information on the nature of the cancer type and the individual patient's treatment plan. Detailed and accurate scans (CT, MRI or PET) will also be used in accurately diagnosing the type of cancer and its extent of spread within the body.

Often sensitive blood tests used to assess cancer activity within the body can be used as a baseline on which to assess the effectiveness of treatment and used to monitor patients after primary treatment has completed. After these investigations have been completed individual patient's case history will be presented at regular multi-disciplinary meetings where the expert specialists discuss the best treatment plan for the individual patient.

Surgery

We are lucky and privileged to work closely with some of the UK's best and most experienced surgeons. Surgeons will often use their professional expertise to remove visible cancer, in the form of an operation. Dependent on the individual patient's disease, these operations can be very small minor procedures with limited impact on the body to very large multi-organ surgery which will have a greater impact on the patient and their quality of life.

Radiotherapy

Radiotherapy is often used in the management of patients with cancer. Often it can be used after surgery to reduce the likelihood of recurrence of the disease. In principle it relies on the fact that human tissue has high water content. It involves directing a beam of high-energy waves (similar to X-rays) to the specified area of the body. These waves cause the water molecules in the tissue to ionise and release strong agents which interfere with the division of the cells, both healthy and cancerous.

As these waves also cause damage to healthy cells and tissue the use of radiotherapy is always planned very carefully, pre-treatment. In the last few years the precision with which radiotherapy can be delivered has had a great impact on the role of radiotherapy in the management of cancer, with such developments as the cyber knife / gamma knife / proton accelerators greatly increasing the number of patients who previously had fewer treatment options for their disease.

Chemotherapy

Chemotherapy was first established as a treatment over fifty years ago and has developed into a sophisticated mechanism of cancer management. As our knowledge of cancer has improved, we have been able to develop drugs which interfere with cancer cell division and disease progression. Chemotherapy uses specific drugs, often in combination, to interfere with cell division at a cellular/microscopic level.

After extensive research and clinical trials to discover the best combinat ion/ frequency of chemotherapy, there are hundreds of different regimes available to the oncologist for the best management of the patient's individual disease.

Principles of Treatment

The treatment for cancer mainly consists of using a combination of different interventions at different times in the individual treatment plan.

Neo-adjuvant: Chemotherapy is often given before surgery to reduce the size or volume of the disease that the surgeon will remove during operation.

Adjuvant: Chemotherapy is given after surgery / radiotherapy for the management of any residual microscopic disease. Adjuvant treatment is often presented as an extra insurance after surgery for the prevention of cancer recurrence.

Palliative Treatment

Cancer sometimes presents in patients to such an extent of disease progression that it is not possible to remove all the cancer as it has spread to other organs in the body, or is impossible to remove surgically. Chemotherapy in this setting is given to minimize disease activity and symptoms and often involves batches of treatment given over a period of time – in many cases, decades.

Types of Chemotherapy

Chemotherapy in a very broad sense can be divided into two main types.

1 Non-cancer cell specific chemotherapy

The different stages in human cell division have been known for many years and chemotherapy drugs have been developed, after extensive research, to interfere with cell division at these different stages. This is why chemotherapy is often given at very specific times in very specific combinations, to best interfere with cell division. However, these drugs will also have an impact on the healthy cells that are continuously dividing and replacing, and often the side effects of chemotherapy are down to the impact that these drugs have on healthy non-cancerous cells.

2 Cancer cell specific chemotherapy

In the last fifteen years, chemotherapy drugs have been developed that target only cancer cells. These often expensive and sophisticated drugs will therefore often minimise the unwelcome side effects of treatment by having no impact on healthy non-cancerous cells. These drugs are currently only available to patients whose cancer type will be sensitive to them and this sensitivity is pre-determined during initial investigations to classify the cancer type.

It is a hope and goal of cancer treatment to further refine and develop new drugs that target just cancer cells specific to the individual. Recent developments in chemotherapy have included drugs that minimise the ability of certain cancer tumours to grow larger than a tiny insignificant cluster of cells.

Chemotherapy protocols often involve a combination of drugs both cancer / and non-cancer cell specific. The decision as to which drugs, doses and frequency relies on the expertise of the oncologist, based on the individual patient.

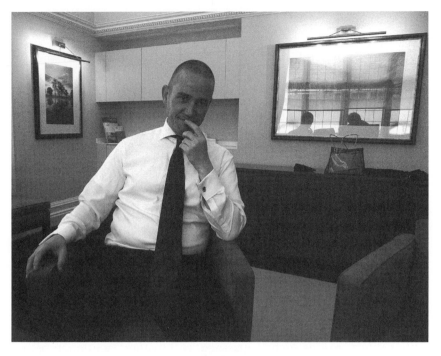

Mike Jones

Common Side Effects of Chemotherapy

Chemotherapy involves the use of strong, often toxic, drugs which have potentially significant side effects. In meeting patients attending the LOC for a pre-chemo assessment these side effects are discussed, and how these effects are best managed.

Blood counts: Human blood is a soup of different types of cells, plasma, salts and minerals. All have a vital role to play in healthy body function. Blood cells are produced in the bone marrow of the long bones of the body and are constantly in production. Some chemotherapy will temporarily interfere with the production of the blood cells, and therefore their levels will drop as a consequence. This effect is often worst felt a few weeks after treatment (a stage often called a Nadir or low stage). One of the specific cells which can be affected are white cells which are cells specific to controlling infection and maintaining the immune system.

This will leave the patient vulnerable for a few days to bacterial infections. It requires careful monitoring of blood counts, observations of symptoms of infection, such as raised temperature, and often includes preventative medications such as growth factor injections to stimulate the body's white cell production. Red cell counts (orhaemaglobin) levels are also closely monitored and are likely to drop as a consequence of treatment.

The other component of blood responsible for clotting is also lowered, meaning that patients on occasion can experience bruising or occasional nose bleeds. Blood counts are carefully monitored throughout treatment and often are maintained or recover with minimal intervention.

Nausea / Vomiting

Chemotherapy drugs are often potent drugs that the body can react to with symptoms of nausea occasionally leading to vomiting. Not all chemotherapy drugs cause nausea, but those classed as having a high risk are used in combination with medicines that minimise the risk of nausea. The drugs are given before and after treatment and are often very successful in minimising the potential of nausea. Other interventions such as massage, reflexology, acupuncture and state of hydration can often be used successfully in the prevention and management of nausea in chemotherapy.

Bowel Habit Changes

Chemotherapy can often cause changes in bowel habit, from causing a mild constipation (often as a result of the anti-sickness medicines) to causing a degree of diarrhoea or loose stool. One of the most important things that a patient can do during chemotherapy is to maintain a good degree of oral fluid intake (approx. 2 litres daily).

By maintaining a good hydration and the use of mild laxatives, or anti-diarrhoeal agents, this will often be enough to manage these temporary changes in bowel habit.

Sensitivity Changes

Some of the chemotherapy drugs can cause an interaction with the nerve cells in the tips of the fingers and toes (peripheral neuropathy). This may sometimes lead to a temporary change in sensitivity in these places. The doses of these drugs are very closely monitored and on occasion these are dose-adjusted, relative to the sensitivity changes felt by the individual patient.

Taste Changes / Mouth Care

Chemotherapy can often lead the patient to experience taste changes or in some cases breakdown of the mouth tissue, presenting in mouth ulcers or tender areas. Mouth care (such as mouthwashes), if used vigilantly, often are all that's required to help minimise these potential side effects. Distorted taste sensations will also recover after treatment has been completed.

Tiredness / Fatigue

This is perhaps the most common side effect of chemotherapy. A majority of patients will be able to maintain a near normal life involving family and work, but will often feel more tired, usually as a progressive symptom based on the more treatment given. Sleep is an important component of chemotherapy as it is often the time that the body does a majority of its healing and recovery. Energy levels will often fluctuate on treatment with better levels at the start and end of each cycle but with worsened levels at the mid-point (nadir).

Hair Loss / Alopecia

A number of the chemotherapy drugs used can potentially cause hair loss by preventing cell division in the hair follicle and causing weakness in the root of the hair, preventing hair growth and causing hair loss. This is an important and significant side effect of treatment and often causes some patients the most concern and anxiety.

In some patients receiving chemotherapy a process called scalp-cooling is used to minimise or even prevent the risk of hair loss. In principle it works by stopping the blood supply to the hair follicle by cooling the scalp to below -5°C. This shuts down the tiny blood vessel feeding the follicle and prevents any of the chemotherapy drugs reaching the follicle, preventing hair loss.

In order for this to work a close-fitting cap (similar to a riding hat) is worn before the administration of the drugs, during the infusion and for a period of time after. All patients have a different tolerance to the discomfort experienced by wearing the cold cap and all decisions regarding its use are individual to the patient. The success of the cold cap relies on different factors, including hair type, strength of drugs used, the tolerance to cooling and luck.

How Chemotherapy Is Given

At present the majority of chemotherapy is given intravenously, that is, into a vein. This delivers the drugs directly into the bloodstream and to the cell. This can be either via a needle which is inserted at each treatment into a vein (peripheralcannula) or via a semi-permanent device called a central line (usually either a portacath or Hickman line). The decision to which type used is often made during the treatment planning.

Certain chemotherapy requires multiple administrations and for a matter of safety is best delivered through a central line. Needle phobia is a very common and appropriate emotion and is best managed with a clinical team very experienced in peripheral IV access and the use of central line devices.

Oral Medications

Recent developments in cancer treatment have provided some new medications available for cancer patients. These include a number of tablet or oral chemotherapy treatments that enable the patient to take regular daily medications at home. Although they do not require IV access they are still very potent drugs, with side effects that require close monitoring. There are also a significant numbers of cancer patients who rely on hormonal therapies (breast/prostate cancer) which are taken as an oral medicine.

The Team

Cancer is a disease which has both a physical and a psychological effect on the patient and close family and friends. In order to provide the best support and care it is often necessary to use a multi-disciplinary team approach in care planning.

So finally, I list the many and varied professional occupations who will all come together as part of that team. All will play their part and are listed at random:

Consultant; Clinic doctor / RMO; nurses / health care assistants; pharmacists / pharmacy technicians; receptionists; medical secretaries; treatment schedulers; patient catering assistants; porters; cleaners; hair and beauty practitioners; complementary therapists; psychologists; psychiatrists; dieticians; and homoeopathists.

The Paxman Cold Caps

MAHDU PARMAR PhD

A friend's five-year-old boy had a brain tumour removed and is receiving chemotherapy. He is extraordinarily brave. His mother sends frequent emails to all friends and parents in her son's class at school. So affected and concerned were the number of boys in his class that when he started to lose his hair they immediately showed their solidarity by having their own heads shaved.

BARONESS KINNOCK OF HOLYHEAD

One of the biggest concerns, when Gemma was finding out about what was going to happen to her over the next few months of cancer treatment, was about losing her hair. Her hair, as for every human being, is visible to everyone though it is dead, but it gives people confidence, individuality and a sense of normality. To have to cope with all the treatments was going to be difficult enough without losing her hair. Gemma was determined and prepared to try anything.

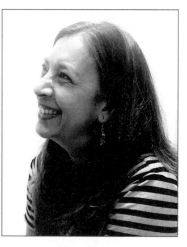

Mahdu Parmar

The solution came in the form of a scalp-cooling device that Gemma would have to spend significant amounts of time under. It required mental and emotional preparation to go through with the constant company of friends. And it was worth it . . . Gemma retained her hair through her whole cancer treatments.

By now, thoughts of writing a book had emerged and the makers of the cooling device had to be included!

It was in May 2011 that we visited Paxman in *Last of the Summer Wine* country, near Huddersfield. There in an ordinary-looking building, a story of entrepreneurship, innovation and a touching humanitarian effort slowly unfolded.

Sue was a confident, very strong and beautiful, thirty-year-old woman with four children (Curtis, Claire, Richard and James) in 1992 when she was diagnosed with breast cancer. She went to a consultant at Huddersfield hospital, Dr Richard Sainsbury, who would become a great family support.

It was very difficult . . . don't make plans for the future, go through the treatment procedures and you will probably lose your hair. The type of cells in cancer, hair and nails rapidly divide so these are affected by chemotherapy, resulting in killing the cancer cells, as well as causing toxicity in hair and nail cells. Scalp-cooling reduces the blood flow to the area and therefore reduces the concentration of cytotoxic drugs reaching the hair follicles during the infusion period. The hospital had a cooling system that they could use to try and prevent Sue losing her hair, but there was no guarantee.

Sue went through the treatment and was positive. She was supported by her husband, Glenn, as well as family and friends. Glenn, an engineer like his father, Eric, who developed and patented ice-bank technology to deliver cellar-chilled beer, was unlikely to have realised the impact it would have on the lives of cancer patients fifty years later.

Sue had surgery to remove her lymph nodes. During her treatment at Huddersfield she had scalp-cooling, a treatment developed thirty years before. The cooling system did not work for Sue. There was a limited history of scalp-cooling. The first method of reducing hair loss was by using a tourniquet followed by ice caps and gel caps at minus 25°C (using the principal of static heat transfer). The ice caps required nurses to top up the ice every twenty minutes, so it was very resource intensive for them. These systems were developed and improved further but still had issues in use, for example leaving bald patches where there was an air pocket under the cooling cap and the scalp was therefore not cooled.

When Sue woke up one morning, she cried out in anguish when finding all her hair was left on the pillow. Until then it was bearable; all the treatments and worries, the children not realising the gravity

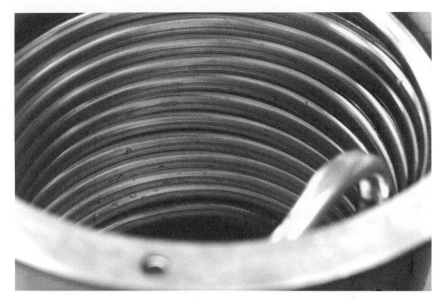

Cooling ingenuity

of the situation. Suddenly, seeing her hair on the pillow was a stark expression of her condition. The impact on everyone, particularly Glenn and the children, was immense. This motivated Glenn to find a better solution for Sue.

Glenn talked to Dr Richard Sainsbury to understand why the cooling system had not worked . . . it was to do with the cooling. Since the family history and expertise was in cooling, how could this acquired knowledge be applied here? Glenn asked his brother Neil to have a look at the system used at Huddersfield.

The temperature varied from minus 5°C to plus 5°C. Over the following years, it became Glenn's and Neil's project. They worked on narrowing the temperature range. Using a cooling temperature of minus 10°C was the optimum, cool enough to prevent hair loss and still remain comfortable for patients.

Glenn had experience and expertise in engineering and business but to improve the head-cooling system he had to learn the principles of medicine and how to develop a medical device where patient safety is paramount. His naivety and determination enabled him to overcome hurdles. Glenn talked to hospital staff from as many hospitals as he could to understand and collect information. He found out how they tried to prevent hair loss; what made it happen; what types of medication caused it; how the patients felt; what the doctors' and nursing staff's attitudes were to hair loss; and much more. He realised that hair loss has a huge impact on patients and the people in their lives, and it was worth focusing on to find a real solution.

It was five years on and Sue was ill with cancer again. The project had been running on the back burner and finding a solution became urgent. Glenn managed to get some money from an investment company to work on the ideas. One of the biggest hurdles was that many oncologists could not see the benefit of scalp-cooling, particularly the emotional benefit. They needed clinical trial information to be convinced of the benefit of yet another treatment for the patient. It was like pushing water uphill. The nursing staff who are much closer to the patient on a day-to-day level were, on the other hand, very supportive and open to trying new approaches to help patients.

In 1995, Sue used an early version of the Paxman scalp cooler. Sadly, Sue passed away, aged forty-four, but her legacy was to gain momentum. The Paxmans were specialists in cooling systems but had no experience of medical devices. They had no clinical data. For their cooling system to be used, it had to go through a full medical regulatory process and gain approval. With the help and support of the Royal Infirmary, Huddersfield Hospital and Dr Richard Sainsbury, they started to develop a clinical data package. The first clinical trial was carried out in 1996.

They also built links with Dr Wim Breed, an oncologist in the Netherlands, who has dedicated his work to scalp-cooling and is president of a foundation called *Geef Haar een Kans* – 'Give hair / her a chance'.

The scalp coolers are made on site. In the workshop are Phillip Haines, a refrigeration engineer, who started working in Brewfitt, the beer-cooling business, in 1992. He started working with Neil in Paxman Coolers to modify the equipment. Scot Hartley has been working in the team for three years and Lucasz Hainc joined one year ago.

All go and service the machines on the ward in hospitals and clinics. They get to see the patients and also talk to them. The team get feedback through the sales team and clinics, and make

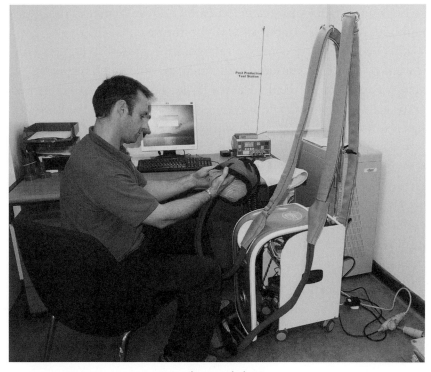

In the workshop

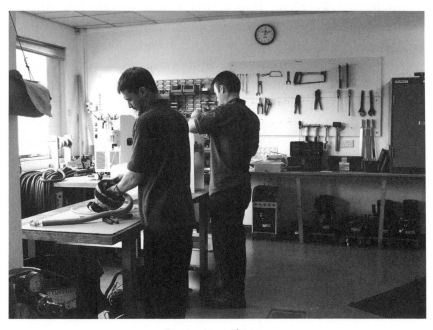

Paxman engineers

improvements and update the machines. Developments to reduce nail toxicity are also underway for the future.

The base unit is a compact refrigeration system which is connected to a specially designed silicone cap. There are five different sizes of caps, extra-small to extra-large, the small cap being red. Caps are also made to suit different-shaped heads. The new system has a softer silicone cap which improves contact with the scalp and is softer on the head. The Paxman aims are always to try to make the caps more comfortable and to offer the best experience for the patient, but also for the nursing staff and doctors.

Originally the coolant in the tank circulated at minus 10°C, reducing the scalp temperature to below 20°C. Development of a new system has allowed a temperature of minus 5°C to be used, which still maintains a scalp temperature of below 20°C and is a lot more comfortable for the patient. A neoprene cover insulates, as well as absorbing any dampness going onto patients. Paxman have a small production facility, producing 250 machines per year. They also carry out service and maintenance on existing machines.

The Orbis I is a one-patient system (mainly used in private hospitals) and the Orbis II is a two-patient system. Having two patients treated at the same time builds patient pairs who meet every time they have their treatment. Currently the NHS has about 700 of the Orbis II in over 300 hospitals in the UK. 1,400 systems have been sold worldwide, mainly in Europe. Paxman are now extending to Japan, South Korea, Russia, South America, the USA and beyond.

Claire tells her mum's story as she visits hospitals. It is a real family business with everyone involved, committed to help people with cancer and keeping Sue's memory alive. They have the passion and determination from a humanitarian point of view to make a difference to patients, families and friends. Their mission is to increase awareness of scalp-cooling worldwide and establish it as a common treatment practice for all patients undergoing chemotherapy.

A campaign to raise awareness was also launched last year called 'Cool Head and Warm Heart', using a picture: a lady with flowers, which is patient focused and families can understand that. Glenn

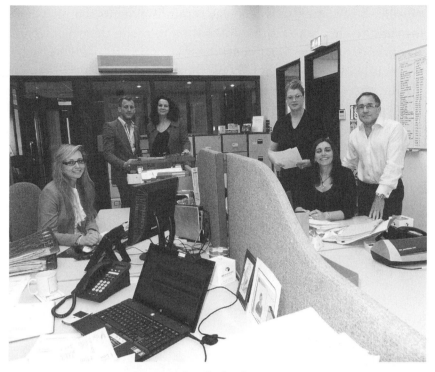

Paxman family business team

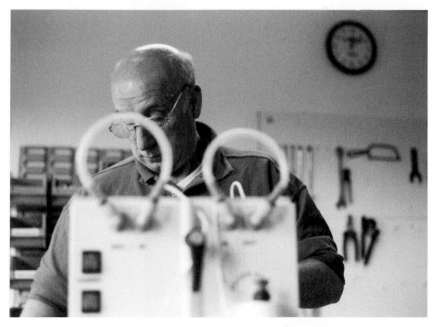

Paxman engineer in workshop

calls her Susie, after his wife. Susie reminds patients that they have the right to choose to have scalp-cooling to retain their dignity and emotion during their treatment.

Recently, donations from 'Walk the Walk', a charity in support of integrated care against breast cancer, has enabled 350 more Paxman scalp-coolers to go to patients in UK hospitals by the end of 2011, and will be able to treat 700 patients per week.

There is good coverage in the UK with oncologists now using the technology as part of the standard treatment. Gemma is doing her part in raising the awareness and supporting the benefits of having a cool head and warm heart during cancer treatment. You can make a difference too . . .

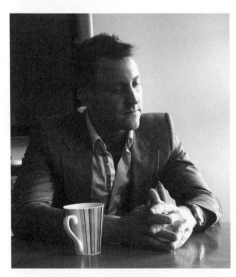

Richard Paxman

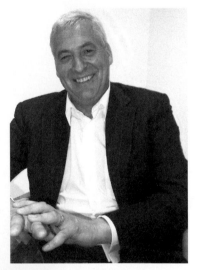

Glenn Paxman: Founder and Chairman

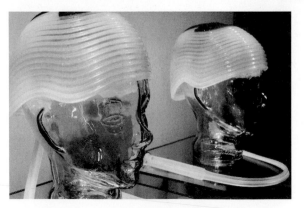

Display Cold Caps

Breast Cancer: The Surgeon's View

PROFESSOR KEFAH MOKBEL MBBS, MS, FRCS
Cosmetic Breast Surgeon

Cancer is a deadly enemy, but its foe – improving medicine – beats its back a little more as each year passes. With sufficient resources, this is a battle that courage and medicine can win.

THE RT HON SIR JOHN MAJOR KG CH ACIB

The Normal Breast

The female breast is made up of fat and milk glands. These glands are composed of basic units called lobules, and are drained by tubes (or ducts) that open at the nipple. The glandular part of the breast is in the middle and feels firmer than the surrounding fatty tissue (Figure 1).

The relative proportions of milk glands, ducts and fat in the breast change with a woman's age and also during pregnancy. For example, the breast of a 25-year-old woman is mainly made up of milk glands, whereas, during pregnancy and breast-feeding, the number of milk glands increases substantially. The female sex hormone oestrogen acts on the breast to maintain the milk glands

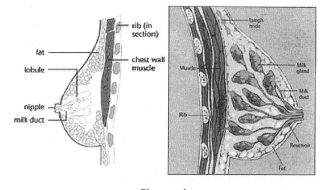

Figure 1

and ducts. During the menopause there is a decrease in the level of this hormone that causes the shrinkage of the glandular part of the breast. The glands are replaced by fat, which is why the breasts often feel softer after the menopause. Hormone replacement therapy helps to prevent these changes (see HRT).

The breast also contains special channels called lymphatic vessels. These vessels transport fluid that accumulates between the cells and return it back into the blood circulation. The lymphatic vessels connect with lymph glands (also called lymph nodes). These are located all over the body. Most of the lymph glands draining the breast are found in the armpit. Cancer cells can spread along lymph vessels and into the lymph glands, causing them to enlarge.

What Is Breast Cancer?

The cell is the basic building block of the body, making up all of our tissues and organs. As cells grow old and wear out, new ones replace them. This process is called cell division, as is illustrated in Figure 2.

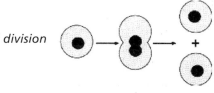

cell division

Figure 2

The balance between dying and growing cells is vital to maintain the normal functioning of our bodies. If the number of growing cells exceeds the number of dying cells, then a lump (or tumour) will develop. If the cells in the tumour divide haphazardly and grow in an aggressive manner, this is called a cancer or malignant tumour.

Malignant cells have the potential of invading adjacent tissues and can spread to other parts of the body some distance away from the main (or primary) tumour. This process of distant spread is called metastasis. It can occur through the blood stream or the lymph vessels.

A breast cancer occurs when the cells of the milk glands or the milk ducts grow and divide in a disorderly manner. This may be detected as a lump in the breast. It can take months or years for a tumour of 1 cm in diameter to grow in the breast. It is estimated that a tumour of this size contains one billion breast cancer cells!

What Are the Different Types of Breast Cancer?

There are two main types of breast cancer: invasive and non-invasive (Table 1).

Type 1 – *Invasive Breast Cancer*

This cancer is more aggressive and has the ability to spread elsewhere in the body and thus cause death.

Type 2 – *Non-invasive Breast Cancer*

This type is confined to the ducts or lobules of the milk glands. It is a non-invasive cancer and does not usually spread to other parts of the body. However, it may develop into an invasive type if left untreated. The medical name for non-invasive breast cancer is ductal carcinoma in situ (DCIS) if it occurs in the milk gland ducts (tubes), or lobular carcinoma in situ (LCIS) if it occurs in the gland lobules.

Breast cancer type		
Details	Invasive	Non-invasive
Behaviour	Aggressive	Not particularly aggressive
Spread	Yes	Not usually
Outcome	Can cause death	Much better prognosis

LCIS is not considered as cancer as such. The presence of this abnormality in a breast biopsy means the patient has an increased risk of developing breast cancer. The risk means that about 1 in 3 women with LCIS will develop breast cancer within 30 years of being diagnosed with the original condition.

Are You at Risk of Getting Breast Cancer?

The risk of developing breast cancer increases with age; an average European woman aged 25 years has a 1 in 15,000 chance of developing breast cancer; for a 40-year-old woman the risk is 1 in 200, for a 50-year-old woman the chance is 1 in 50, and at the age of 80 years the chance is 1 in 11.

The number of cases of breast cancer is five times higher in Western countries than in Far Eastern countries such as Japan and China. However, Japanese women who move to the USA increase their risk of developing breast cancer, which shows that the environment also plays an important role.

Risk factors are things that increase your chance of developing breast cancer. The main groups are shown in Table 2.

1 Cancer history	2 Hormonal	3 Lifestyle	4 Other
Family history	Age when periods started	Obesity after the menopause	Environment
Previous breast cancer	Age at first pregnancy	Diet	Breast biopsy
	Age at menopause	Alcohol	
	Use of 'the pill'		
	Use of HRT		

Cancer History Risk Factors

Family History of Breast Cancer

It is thought that up to 5 per cent of all breast cancers are inherited owing to the presence of abnormal genes. These genes are passed on from mother to daughter, so having a first-degree relative (such as a sister or mother) with breast cancer will increase your chance of developing the disease. This is particularly true if the relative develops breast cancer in both her breasts, or before she reaches the age of 45 years. A family history of breast cancer in a first-degree male relative is also associated with a significant increase in breast cancer risk. Breast cancer in a distant relative has little effect on your breast cancer risk.

Your chance of developing breast cancer doubles if one first-degree relative developed the disease before the age of 45 years. If two first-degree relatives developed the disease before the age of 45 years, then your chance of developing breast cancer is four times greater than normal.

Scientists have identified several genes responsible for transmitting breast cancer. Three of the most important of these breast cancer genes are called BRCA-1, BRCA-2 and P53. This inherited form of breast cancer usually develops before the age of 50 years. If a woman has not developed breast cancer by the age of 50 years, despite having a first-degree relative with breast cancer, it is unlikely that she carries the abnormal gene(s).

The BRCA-1 gene is also associated with ovarian cancer. So, the presence of other types of cancer, such as cancer of the womb or ovary, in addition to breast cancer, also suggests the possibility that there is a cancer-causing gene in the family. Testing for breast cancer genes is now possible, but may require the presence of living relatives who have had breast cancer, and it may also take a long time to identify the gene.

A significant family history of prostate cancer (early age of onset before the age of 55, more than one relative) is also associated with an increased risk of breast cancer.

Cancer of the Other Breast
This increases the likelihood of breast cancer in the remaining breast.

Hormonal Risk Factors

Starting Periods Before the Age of 11 Years
Women who have a history of starting their periods (menses) before the age of 11 have a higher chance of developing breast cancer. This is thought to be due to their longer exposure to the female sex hormone oestrogen, which is an established risk factor for breast cancer.

Later Pregnancy
The risk of developing breast cancer increases by 5 per cent for each year of delay in having the first full-term pregnancy. Women who have their first child before the age of 30 have a lower risk of developing breast cancer than those whose first pregnancy occurs after the age of 35. Recent research indicates that breast-feeding also reduces the risk of developing breast cancer.

There is no scientific evidence that pregnancies which end in a spontaneous or induced miscarriage increase the risk of developing breast cancer.

Later Menopause

The average age of a woman upon reaching the menopause in western Europe is 50. Women who reach the menopause after the age of 53 have a higher chance of developing breast cancer. Delayed menopause prolongs a women's exposure to oestrogen – just as does starting periods before the age of 11.

The Oral Contraceptive Pill

The taking of the oral contraceptive pill that contains oestrogen within the previous ten years slightly increases the chance of developing breast cancer. The greater the oestrogen-content in the pill, the higher the risk of developing breast cancer. Again, this is because oestrogen increases the risk of breast cancer. However, breast cancer that develops in contraceptive pill users seems to be less advanced than in non-users.

Hormone Replacement Therapy (HRT)

Taking HRT after the menopause seems to increase the risk of developing breast cancer, especially if it is continued for more than ten years.

HRT, however, reduces the risk of brittle-bone disease (osteoporosis), bone fractures and large bowel cancer. It also improves the symptoms of the menopause, such as vaginal dryness, hot flushes and depression. It is currently thought that HRT should be avoided where possible in women with a personal or a significant family history of breast cancer. A recent American study (Women's Health Initiative) has shown that taking HRT increases the risk of breast cancer and coronary heart disease. Therefore the author believes that the benefit-risk balance for HRT is negative and that the lowest dose should be used for the shortest time if required.

Lifestyle Risk Factors

Obesity

Obesity after the menopause increases the risk of breast cancer in women, whereas obesity before the menopause seems to reduce breast cancer risk. In post-menopausal women the body fat is the main source of oestrogen production; so obese women will have more oestrogen on board, thus increasing their breast cancer risk.

(The main source of oestrogen production in pre-menopausal women is the ovaries.)

Diet

The research studies looking at the issue of diet and breast cancer show conflicting results. However, it is thought that a high intake of saturated animal fats and red meat (especially if overcooked) increases the risk of developing breast cancer, whereas diets high in fibre and vitamins (A, C and E), such as fresh fruits and vegetables, decrease the risk. It is also thought that fish and green tea reduce the risk of breast cancer.

Alcohol Consumption

Recent evidence suggests that excessive alcohol intake increases the likelihood of breast cancer. The risk seems to increase with all types of alcoholic drinks.

Smoking

There is increasing evidence that both active and passive smoking increase the risk of breast cancer especially in women younger than 50 years.

There is no evidence that the personal use of hair-dyes increases breast cancer risk.

Other Risk Factors

The Environment

Earlier we said that Japanese women who had moved to the USA developed a similar breast cancer risk to that of the American population. This indicates that there are powerful environmental factors influencing the risk of developing breast cancer. Apart from diet and life-style, certain chemicals, such as pesticides, are thought to increase the risk. As yet, there is no established evidence to support this link. Exposure to radiation also increases the risk of many cancers, including breast cancer.

It is important to realise that the radiation dose used in mammography (X-rays of the breast) is too small to be a significant risk factor.

Previous Benign Breast Biopsy

The risk of breast cancer is not significantly increased if you have had a previous breast biopsy (surgical) for a benign condition, such a cyst or a simple fibroadenoma. However, the presence of certain microscopic features in a breast biopsy is associated with a higher risk. For example, the risk is increased by 4–5 times if a condition known as atypical epithelial hyperplasia is found in the breast biopsy.

Mammographic Density

Mammographic density in 75 per cent or more of the breast is associated with an almost five-fold increased risk of breast cancer, and this risk persists for an extended period of time. In addition, for women with extensively dense breasts, the masking effect of dense breast tissue increases the odds more than 17 times of a cancer being missed and then detected by non-screening methods. In such cases the addition of ultrasound scan and MRI imaging to digital mammography should be considered.

The risk factors are summarised in Table 3.

What Does 'Increased Risk' Mean to You?

Understandably, women can become very anxious when they are told that they have an increased risk of developing breast cancer. It should be remembered that the normal risk of breast cancer for a woman aged 30–50 years is 1 in 1000 per year. If your risk were to double it would be 1 in 500 per year; in other words, one woman in every 500 would develop breast cancer within one year.

Risk factor	Increase in risk of breast cancer
Age	x 10 (in the very elderly)
Family history	x 2–9
Country	x 5 (in Western countries)
Cancer in the other breast	x 5
Early menses (before 11 years)	x 3
Late pregnancy (1st child after 40 years)	x 3
Late menopause (after 53 years)	x 2
Obesity after the menopause	x 2
Contraceptive pill (4+ years when young)	x 2
Social Class I & II	x 2
Radiation	x 1.5–3.0
Previous benign breast biopsy	x 1.5
HRT (10+ years)	x 1.5
High alcohol intake	x 1.1-2.0

How Can You Reduce the Risk?

The good news is that some of the risk factors mentioned in the previous section can be modified to reduce the risk of breast cancer.

General Lifestyle

- Avoid becoming overweight after the menopause.
- Undertake regular exercise and increase physical activity (min. 1 hour per week).
- Avoid excessive alcohol intake – try not to drink more than 6 units of alcohol per week (equivalent to one glass of wine per day).
- Reduce the intake of animal fat and red meat (esp. overcooked red meat).
- Eat more fish (excluding farmed salmon).
- Replace full-fat dairy products with low-fat dairy products
- Increase the intake of fresh fruits and vegetables, especially: cranberries, raspberries, cherries, red grapes and pomegranates. These fruits can be also taken as fresh juice drinks with no added artificial ingredients (e.g. fresh smoothies).
- Increase the intake of green tea.
- Increase the intake of olive oil.

Comment: There is no credible scientific evidence that underarm cosmetics and low-fat dairy products increase the risk of developing breast cancer. Soya products seem to be neutral, that is, they cause neither harm nor benefit regarding breast cancer.

Hormonal

- Avoid taking HRT after the menopause and try to use alternatives to HRT.
- Try to have your first child before the age of 30 and avoid pregnancy after the age of 40.

Other Ways (for Women at High Risk)

- Anti-oestrogen drugs, such as Tamoxifen (a breast cancer drug) and raloxifene (used to protect post-menopausal women from developing osteoporosis), have been shown to reduce the risk of breast cancer by 50–75 per cent. However, further research is needed before these drugs can be recommended for breast cancer prevention.
- Preventative mastectomy (removal of the whole breast) seems

to reduce the risk of breast cancer by 90 per cent in high-risk women, such as those who carry breast cancer genes. Preventive oophorectomy also decreases the risk of developing breast cancer in BRCA-1 and BRCA-2 gene carriers.

- Recent research suggests that aspirin-like drugs may reduce the risk of developing breast cancer. Further research is needed before these drugs can be recommended for breast cancer prevention.
- A new breast cancer drug called Arimidex has been found to be better than Tamoxifen in preventing breast cancer in the opposite breast among post-menopausal women with breast cancer, but further research is needed.

The author believes that the following dietary measures may also reduce the risk of breast cancer:

- Increased consumption of antioxidants. These include the vitamins A, C and E, and the minerals selenium, zinc and sulphur. They are found in fresh fruit and vegetables.
- Increased intake of fibre. It is thought that a high-fibre diet may reduce the breast cancer risk by binding dietary oestrogen (present in food) in the bowel and preventing it from being absorbed into the blood stream. Fibre is plentiful in cereals, brown bread, fruits and vegetables.
- Reduced intake of animal fat and red meat. Replace red meat with fish – it is a good source of protein and antioxidants. If you do eat red meat, try to avoid over-cooking it.
- Increased intake of red cherries, grapes and green tea.

Breast Screening

What is the Purpose of Breast Screening?
The aim of breast screening is to detect breast cancer at an early stage in women who appear well and do not have any symptoms of the disease. The earlier breast cancer is detected, the more likely it is to be treatable.

The screening methods currently used include:

- Self-examination of the breasts;
- Breast examination by a doctor;
- Mammography (breast X-ray).

Breast self-examination (Figure 3) may be performed every month, preferably at the same point in the menstrual cycle, for example, five days after the last day of the your period. Follow these steps when performing self-examination:

(a) Stand up in front of a mirror with your arms down by your sides. Make sure that the room has good lighting.

(b) Look for any changes in the basic appearance of your breasts, such as puckering of the skin, in-drawing of the nipple, or enlargement of one breast.

(c) Repeat this with your arms raised above your head – this will make certain abnormalities more obvious.

(d) Next, lie flat on your back on a firm, comfortable surface, such as a bed. Using the flat parts (pads) of your fingers to feel your breasts, begin with the right hand examining the left breast, and the left hand examining the right breast.

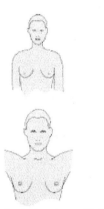

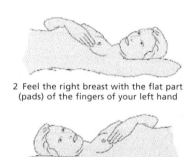

2 Feel the right breast with the flat part (pads) of the fingers of your left hand

3 Examine the left breast with your right hand

1 Stand in front of a mirror with the arms down and then raised above the head

Breast self-examination

(e) Move your fingers in a circular motion and examine each quarter of the breast. Remember that the breast extends up to the collarbone and across into the armpit – so examine these areas too. (Remember that the lymph glands draining the breasts are located in the armpits, and breast cancer may spread to these glands, causing their enlargement.)

Breast Examination by a Doctor

If you discover any changes, consult your doctor! His examination of your breasts will involve going through similar steps.

Mammography (Breast X-ray)

Mammography is a way of imaging the breast tissue and produces an X-ray called a mammogram. The breast is 'squashed' between two plastic plates while a beam of X-rays passes through the breast tissue and on to an X-ray film. This 'squashing' of the breast may be a little uncomfortable, but it only lasts for approximately 30 seconds. The radiation doses used during mammography are much too small to be significant in causing cancer.

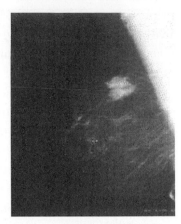

Breast X-ray

The mammogram appears as a mixture of white, grey and black shadows that can be interpreted by a specialist doctor, called a radiologist. Mammograms are 85 per cent accurate in the diagnosis of breast cancer.

Scientific studies in western Europe have shown that breast cancer screening with mammography has reduced the number of deaths from breast cancer by approximately 30 per cent. This applies only to women aged over 50, because mammograms are less likely to show cancers in younger women (with dense breasts). Breast cancers detected by screening are usually at an early stage or are non-invasive cancers that can be treated more effectively.

Screening programmes in countries such as the UK offer mammography to women aged 50–65 once every three years. It is now believed this is too long an interval to go between breast screens, and it is the author's opinion that women aged between 50 and 69 should have a mammogram every two years and that women aged 40–49 should be screened by digital mammography every year. Digital mammography is more accurate that analogue mammography in breast cancer detection, especially in premenopausal women and those taking HRT. Furthermore it allows the use of a low radiation dose. For more information on this topic: http://www.issoonline.com/content/3/1/4

Women with a strong family history of breast cancer are advised to have screening digital mammography every 18 months from the age of 35. As mentioned earlier, younger women (below 35) tend to

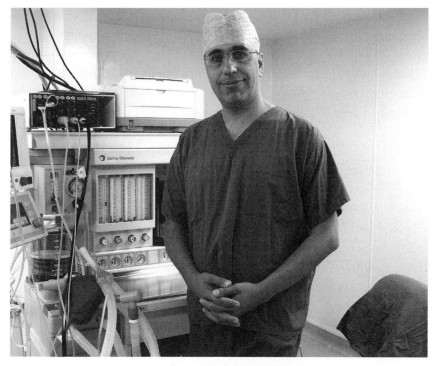

Professor Kefah Mokbel

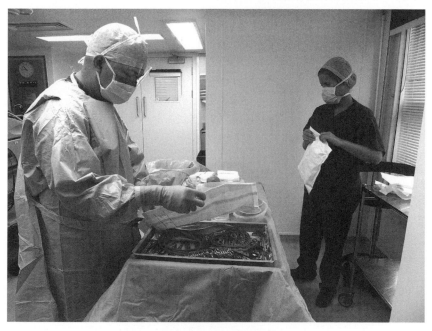

Preparing the operation theatre

have denser breasts and, therefore, the mammogram may not show any abnormal shadows as clearly as in older women. Current research is trying to find better methods of screening younger women, such as magnetic resonance imaging (MRI) and ultrasound scan. Recent evidence strongly suggests that MRI is the best method of screening high-risk younger women.

What Happens if You Have an Abnormal Mammogram?

If the mammogram does show a suspicious shadow, the woman will be recalled to the clinic and examined by a breast specialist. Further tests may be required; these include a needle biopsy of the breast and / or an ultrasound scan.

The tests may reveal that there is a breast lump corresponding to the abnormal shadow on the mammogram. Occasionally, no further tests will be required and the patient will be advised to have a follow-up mammogram in a year, or to continue in the screening programme. If the biopsy shows that cancer cells are present, the patient is treated accordingly.

Breast Augmentation

Reasons for Wanting Bigger Breasts

The first breast enlargement in medical history took place over 100 years ago. The reasons for wanting bigger breasts vary but the main reasons a woman wants breast enlargement are that

- She feels her breasts are too small;
- She has unequal breasts;
- She wants to regain the size and shape of her breasts after pregnancy / breastfeeding or experiencing significant weight loss.

Improvement in body image usually leads to enhanced self-esteem and personal confidence.

Always remember that if you decide to have breast augmentation please make sure you are doing it for yourself and not for others.

The Nurses' Perspective

GWYNEDD BURGOYNE & ANNE ANDERSON
Clinical Nurses, London Breast Institute

Cancer remains the most dreaded word any of us expects to hear from a doctor's lips. Thank God, though, it has often proved to be a containable adversary: in fact, I have lost count of the number of my women friends who have had breast cancer, beaten it and virtually forgotten that they have ever had it. Early detection, swift reaction and loving support in many cases reduce it to a temporary inconvenience, but the relief on all sides is intense and joyous. Life goes on.

SIMON CALLOW CBE

As breast care nurse specialists at the London Breast Institute at the Princess Grace Hospital, we are in a unique position to address many of the needs of our patients throughout screening, diagnosis, treatment and follow-up of benign breast disease, and also breast

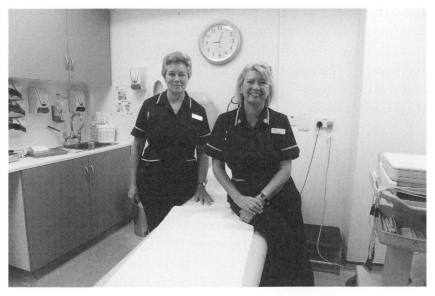

Gwynedd Burgoyne and Anne Anderson

cancer. We have a very different and varied role, compared to the role of clinical nurses on the ward. We are more actively involved in providing essential support and information to empower a woman with breast disease to participate in treatment decisions and take more control over her health and life challenges. However, when clinical intervention is required our practical nursing expertise is utilised.

It has been acknowledged that women with breast cancer and their families embark on a roller coaster ride and the grief and loss embedded in this journey are immense, often exposing the limitations of any coping strategies. We understand completely how difficult and frightening it is for patients to grasp the implications of a breast cancer diagnosis. After receiving the news from the consultant, part of our role is to help the patients comprehend and to assist them in understanding all the treatment options available to them. We are passionate about providing the psychological support and continuity of care throughout the patient's journey and to empower them particularly when treatment choices and decisions need to be made.

When patients speak with us for the first time they will learn that we will be their 'one-stop' resource. We will take the time to get to know them on a personal level which will help us to identify their needs. In order to meet those needs we can help them access appropriate services and answer their questions. We are available to the patient through all the stages of diagnosis, treatment and survivorship. The relationship between us and the patient is personal and will vary, depending on the level of involvement that they and their family require.

Due to the unpredictability and uniqueness of the breast cancer journey, many people oscillate back and forth between stages of their treatment. One seemingly minor event may catapult them backwards into the full force of grief at any one time. Often, real grief is misunderstood: a common complaint heard is: 'No one understands what I am really going through,' or: 'Am I going to die?' and then inevitably, the question: 'What happens now?' These questions are all natural and we are there every step of the way, using our knowledge and expertise to assess and determine the help the patients require to deal with their diagnosis.

We are able to supply the majority of information necessary to understand the nature of the disease, treatment options, possible side effects and strategies for psychological adjustment. This is a highly complex task which requires the breast care nurse to possess well-developed communication skills, expert specialist knowledge and an understanding of the patient's decision-making choices. We oversee and organise the appointments requested for scans and tests that are required in the pre-operative phase and when further scanning is deemed necessary. We also co-ordinate theatre bookings and ensure pre-operative assessment of the patient is documented.

The provision of consistent, clear, tailored information is regarded as the responsibility of all members of the multidisciplinary team but can become blurred when chemotherapy and radiotherapy treatment begins, and the patient meets up with other teams of specialists. We do not hesitate to confer with other members of the multidisciplinary team to ensure that women with breast cancer receive the individualised support and continuity of care they deserve.

Our role is very fulfilling and personally rewarding.

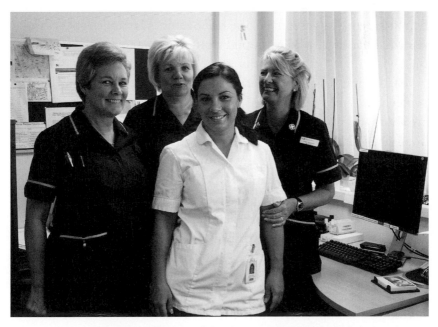

A nursing team at the Princess Grace Hospital

Lymphoedema: Remedial Massage

BERNIE MARTIN

Remedial Massage for Cancer and Lymphodema

I know so many women, friends and family, who have had breast cancer. The majority of them are still alive and well. It proves that medical science is improving all the time, but more importantly that the human spirit is indomitable.

ANGELA RIPPON OBE

I mentioned in my introduction that I had met some extraordinary people along the way who had enriched my life by their skills, integrity and devotion. Bernie Martin is one of them.

After my operation and treatment in radiotherapy, my right arm was swollen and felt heavy. It had also hardened and I was in pain. I went to see my surgeon, Professor Mokbel, who advised that I had lymphoedema and referred me to Bernie Martin, a specialist in remedial massage, who he hoped would be able to reduce the excess fluid which had built up in my arm.

My first impressions of Bernie were positive. He knew what the problem was and how to deal with it. He manipulated the affected areas and was able to reassure me with sympathetic explanation. An hour or so later, the arm swelling had reduced, my movements were again agile and the pain diminished. 'Therapeutic touch' is very important in all healing work, to boost people's confidence and for calming and, of course, to transfer positive energies.

Bernie explained: 'Oedema is an abnormal accumulation of fluid in the body tissues, which can be either localised or general. There are various types and causes of oedema. One of the most common is injury damaging the capillaries (including surgery) which allows fluid to leak out of them, thus flooding the body tissues and causing swelling. The capillaries normally exude and re-absorb the fluid to and from the body tissues in a balanced way. Blockage or removal of lymph nodes of course affects drainage and can result in lymph-oedema, which we try to help as soon as possible using various drainage techniques.'

Bernie said that insurance companies very stupidly refuse to fund an effective therapy which would get patients off their books more quickly, thus saving them money . . . certainly more quickly than just straight physiotherapy, which they do fund! Logic never seems to apply for them. In their ignorance they see the word "massage" and just think of the skin polishing that one would receive at a health spa or from a beauty therapist, rather than treatment for specific conditions.'

Since I have had weekly ongoing treatment, I have learnt a little of the man. My first shock was from one of the nurses at the hospital who told me that Bernie was due for retirement shortly. I was saddened that I might lose a true professional, just when I felt comfortable under his expertise. The following visit, I quietly studied his face.

It is a kind, strong face with humour and compassion that has seen a great deal of life. I thought he did not look sixty-five years old, he looked much younger. Had they made a mistake?

'Bernie, when are you going to retire?' I asked. He replied, 'I don't know, I am only seventy-seven. I'll retire when I *have* to and even then, probably not completely. I hate the thought of not doing anything productive.'

For fifteen years he was in the RAF Medical Service and was also a musician. After leaving the RAF, he played jazz saxophone and piano in some of the famous night clubs in the West End of London. Nowadays, since the night clubs disappeared, he plays the organ in his local church. Throughout his life he had managed both music and remedial and sport massage. He says, 'I thoroughly enjoy working with both. Each rewarding in its own way and there is a definite connection between music and healing.'

I asked Bernie what encouraged him to specialise in cancer.

'I was gradually drawn into it over the years,' he said, 'with the spur of my wife dying with cancer, a long time ago. I feel in a way I'm getting revenge for that, by helping to fight it and treating the after effects when the doctors and surgeons have done their work.'

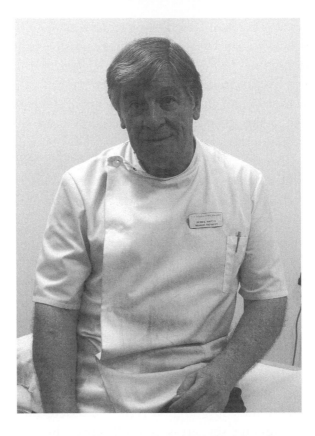

Bernie Martin and below Bernie's hands

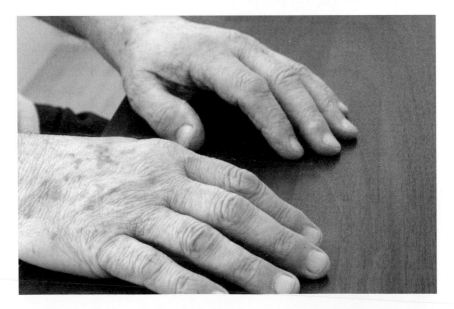

As my right arm is still frail I found I could not hold my heavy Leica camera to proceed with my photographic work.

I asked Bernie, 'When will I be able to lift my camera again?'

He said, 'It's hard to say, everybody is different, but I think that after a reasonable amount of treatment over the next few weeks, we should have your camera back in your hands.'

Yes, for the purpose of this book I did try to use my old-fashioned Leica to work with. My arm tired easily so I was forced to buy a small digital camera, a LUMIX, Panasonic DMC-LX5 with a Leica lens.

The photographs in this book are taken only with this camera. I chose black and white images, as opposed to colour. For a serious book, black and white, it has to be. I have put my Hasselblad and Leica cameras in the cupboard to use for my next book, perhaps?

The National Health:
Two Doctors' Perspectives

We have all been touched by cancer – it is a relentless enemy but not unbeatable. If we fight it together we will rid our world of this terrible disease. Sir Cliff Richard

DR S. NAZEER

The initial presentation was during a routine NHS clinic – coughs, colds, painful knees, aching backs, etc.: a matter-of-fact introduction explaining that she had probably bruised her right breast lifting boxes during her recent move. The breast was tender, very red, hot and swollen and certainly looked as if it had been knocked hard. Other than sending her to the local A&E Department where she would be seen by non-specialist personnel, usual NHS referral, even in suspected cancer, has the possibility of up to a two-week wait. This was not acceptable to her and I wanted her seen as soon as possible.

Fortunately, she was covered by a medical insurance policy which allowed private referrals and care. Half an hour later, she was being examined by one of the UK's top breast specialists. His apprehensions, misconceptions and miscommunications seemed to be the order of the day, regardless of whether these early difficult days are in the public or the private domain. The GP can, and must, make and take time to listen, explain, clear up, dispel, reassure and, above all, care.

Once a clear plan has been set out and roles allocated and recognised, the daily management takes place relatively smoothly. Relatives, friends and the GP fill the gaps of knowledge and uncertainty.

Common to the NHS and the private health care system is the necessary attribute of empathetic care, but both systems rely on human skill and expertise and it is not uncommon for lapses of communication, concern and forethought to occur. Also, resources and facilities can be variable. The atmosphere and space in the private hospitals have been planned and developed particularly well. The NHS tends to have the same concept, but finds imagination and creativity seem to be in short supply. A pleasant space, with a specifically designed chair / bed, provision of comfort and efficient personnel are and should be the basic requirements.

Communication between the specialists, the patient and the GP must be appropriate and detailed. This is person-specific and can cause undue harm and pain if the individual concerned is unthinking and matter of fact. Having a problem with her breast (with all the connotations and apprehensions), the initial consultation with the specialist is especially important and crucial. The denouement needs to be considered, considerate and with enough detail and explanation to inform, but leave the door open for questions and queries later.

Fortunately, her NHS GP was supportive with time, explanation and reassurance. Not all specialists behave inappropriately and not all specialists behave inappropriately all the time!

Equally, not all GPs have the resources necessary to be so much a part of a patient's journey.

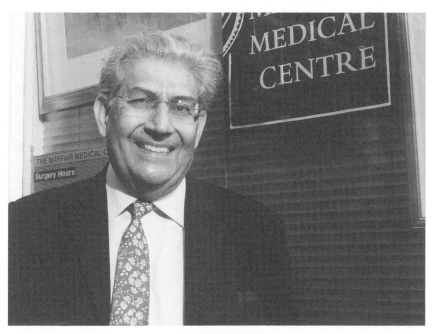

Dr S. Nazeer

We can all help beat the odds of this disease by encouraging those we care about to go to their GP at the very first sign of any symptoms and to take full advantages of the NHS's screening programme. I hope Gemma's book will inspire others facing breast cancer to tackle the challenges ahead.

BORIS JOHNSON

DR J. MOORE

As a doctor I try to always empathise with being in the place of the patient in front of me. The courage it can take to make an appointment, the intense impact that a potentially serious diagnosis can have and the great uncertainty and anxiety this can bring. In every sense, each patient has a unique journey to the clinic or surgery . . . the time before in the waiting room can seem endless.

Meeting a doctor for the first time can have compelling implications for the patient. Psychological research shows that initially patients have four key questions of their new doctor:

(1) Will he listen?
(2) Does he care?
(3) Will he understand what needs to be done?
(4) Will he actually do it?

Evidence shows that patients spend the first 60–90 seconds of the consultation assessing these factors. If the doctor can quickly reassure the patient of these issues very early in a consultation, all will go well; if not, it could be very difficult. Key consultation skills are essential at the beginning, including active listening, empathy and summarising the doctor's understanding of the problem back to the patient early. These are powerful tools in achieving rapid and mutual understanding of the patient's agenda and as the basis for a successful rest of the consultation.

The accurate formulation of a problem lies at the very heart of the art of clinical medicine. Breast cancer is an excellent example of the way doctors prioritise their thoughts in making a diagnosis of cancer.

When any woman presents with a breast lump, easily the most

important factor is the age of the patient. The National Institute for Clinical Excellence (NICE) published *Suspected Cancer Guidelines* in 2005. This states that less than 2 per cent of breast cancers occur in women aged less than 35 and are very rare in women aged less than 30.

Many young women in their teens or early twenties present with firm, round, rubbery lumps called fibroadenoms, or a more diffuse variation called fibroadenosis. Although patients are always understandably anxious, these lumps are almost invariably benign and you can be reassuring. However, at the other end of the spectrum, if a woman in her late seventies or older presents with a breast lump, it is highly likely to be cancerous and therefore must be treated with the utmost caution. Several times in my career I have been faced with very harrowing late onset presentations of advanced breast cancers in older patients.

The next most important factor is the duration of symptoms. For cancer this is often very difficult as patients suddenly become aware of a problem. This is never more common than with breast cancer where a lump is suddenly discovered and the patient will not know how long it has been there. The NICE *Guidance for Suspected Cancer* with respect to breast cancer is very helpful. Women presenting after the menopause, with a lump with suspicious features, need to be referred immediately. For women before the menopause, it is best to monitor until after the next period to assess if changes might be due to hormonal influence; before making a referral. Another important benign cause of breast lumps are breast cysts. These are smooth, round lumps full of fluid. These can be diagnosed with ultrasound and easily drained with a fine needle. If they recur, or are very large, they can be removed surgically.

Another key factor is family history as some breast cancers have a strongly genetic basis. For example in my own family, both my mother and maternal grandmother suffered breast cancer at an early age, putting my sister at significantly increased risk. Families with a strong family history can have genetic screening and then chose pre-emptive surveillance to catch the disease early if they are at risk.

The next stages involve key questions, and then pertinent physical examination findings which help a physician formulate the likelihood that a lesion in the patient's breast is more or less likely to be cancerous. This is a matter of process (guidelines can help you judge the risk more objectively), experience and clinical judgement.

Cancer is of course the most feared diagnosis of all and many patients presenting will expect the worst. Much of our time is spent with conditions which are almost certainly benign and the skill is to reassure. However, it is sometimes daunting when a clinical picture begins to emerge, where a diagnosis of cancer becomes increasingly likely. Trying to achieve that subtle balance between being truthful about your fears, while asserting that further investigation is required to properly establish the cause and the hope and encouragement the patient will need in facing this process.

However, for me the key impact is the moment a patient is told that they have cancer. There is no easy way to do this and the reactions can be intense and varied. Suddenly the patient is faced with a new and very different world immediately opening up before them, full of questions and uncertainty. I hope that the major value of this book is to give answers to these questions from a very special lady who has travelled this journey ahead of you.

Through words and, more powerfully, images, Gemma can share her insight into the road that lies ahead through her great skill in capturing the essence of a moment or explaining a difficult concept through remarkable photography. She has undertaken photographic projects for over forty years, but always as an outsider. For the first time she presents this book from her own very personal experience – as a gift to her fellow patients who are following behind and with an empathy as to what is most important to you.

It is a book for everyone, from all backgrounds and every walk of life. For most of you the questions will be the same:

What does a radiotherapy machine look like?
How and where am I given chemotherapy and what does it involve?
Are there ways to avoid losing my hair?
How can I avoid or minimise the side effects of treatment?
Most importantly, who are the different professionals who will
 be caring for me and what are their roles and skills?

I hope that this book can give really practical and supportive answers to these vital questions which are so immediately important

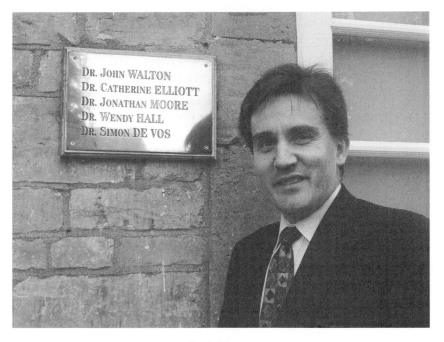

Dr J. Moore

to that person who has suddenly and unexpectedly come face to face with cancer. A first-hand perspective of these essential challenges; addressing the issues through text, photographs and most pertinently through Gemma's own experience, is a much cherished companion at the start of this journey.

The most important theme that should come from this book is hope, encouragement and inspiration to the reader. Cancer treatments have never been better and outcomes continue to improve year by year. The most unforeseen consequence, for Gemma, of becoming a cancer patient has been the extraordinary experiences it has involved. Suddenly thrown into a completely new world, she has met the most exceptional people whom she would have never otherwise encountered. Many of those involved in cancer care are highly inspirational with a real passion to conquer this complex disease, but also devote themselves with real kindness and compassion for every aspect of the care they give.

In September 2011 Matthew Taylor from the Royal Society of Arts published an observational study which clearly concluded that prognosis and outcomes in cancer were very strongly influenced by the degree to which the patients themselves consciously took control of the management of their disease and were actively involved in all aspects of their care. This book is therefore extremely timely in encouraging patients to achieve exactly this and its experiences and insights will be a tremendous support and inspiration.

So the cancer journey – like the essence of life itself – is a complex mix of very strong conflicting emotions. As Professor Daniel Hochhauser so pertinently concludes in his Foreword to this book, it is the empowerment of patients to achieve their optimal healing, in whatever form and extent this takes, as well as encouraging full and active personal involvement in all aspects of their care, which in modern cancer treatments allows patients to find, for themselves, their own pathway back to wholeness.

To the Newly Diagnosed: A Psychological View

DR SUE GESSLER PhD AFBPsS
Clinical Psychologist

I can only admire those I know who have been diagnosed with cancer. They have lived bravely and cheerfully; savouring the preciousness of each moment even more than they did before, and coped somehow with the uncertainty of it all. Are there perhaps more untapped, unexpected inner resources within all of us than we are normally aware of?

PROFESSOR LORD (RICHARD) HARRIES OF PENTREGARTH

Go with the Flow is the title of this book. It is in the imperative form, but really expresses a way of being that has emerged from Gemma's own experience. In some ways, it is a description of the end of a process, but a very personal one.

You will have your own journey – and your own process – and your own way of navigating your journey may be a very different one from Gemma's. It is the aim of this chapter to let you know a range of ideas and resources that exists and that you can choose to use, or not, as you please, with the hope that you can travel these stormy waters and come to your own safe harbour in time.

Many people go through this very difficult experience, but only in retrospect make sense of what was happening at an emotional level. Often they are exposed to many theories, convictions and advice about what they should be doing both physically and mentally.

Cancer is a trauma; its context is the person you were before your diagnosis and the life you were leading. Much of what you are doing on a psychological level is adjusting to the attack on the life you were leading before, the loss of plans you had, or losses occasioned by the treatment; and accommodating to the life you have during and after treatment, with all its unwelcome aspects.

How you navigate this readjustment will be coloured by your general approach to life. Effects of surgery; chemotherapy and its side-effects; and the non-specific but wearing problems such as fatigue – that term which sounds so delicate and benign and is surprising and debilitating and utterly confusing to the sort of person who deals with most problems in their life by being active, for example.

And this is where issues about attitude come in. The world is full of self-help literature from a range of perspectives; exercise, diet, meditation. It's very intriguing to a psychologist in the world of health and medicine that cancer, of all diseases, seems to attract the strongest opinions and imprecations to those who have it. And the existence of a research literature in the field makes this seem more imperative to the patient.

When I first began working in cancer, one of my standard questionnaires to patients at the beginning of treatment included a question on what they believed the causes of their disease to be. Without exception, the top three reasons always included stress. This can be a way of seeing the cancer as an attack from outside; but is also a significant self-blaming view and can be recruited by people to attack themselves still further when they are going through extremely difficult times. It is true that being hopeful is helpful to managing the vicissitudes of treatment; but if you are *not* feeling hopeful and optimistic, it can be even more depressing to be surrounded by people telling you that you *must* think positively, and if you don't you will interfere with your treatment, your cancer will return sooner . . . and so on. I have had a patients say to me that they would like to continue their sessions with me after they went into remission – but they couldn't possibly voice any fears or negative thoughts, as this would cause their chemotherapy to fail and in remission, cause their cancer to return sooner. This is a complex issue; the research literature is still in ferment about what impact psychological and social factors – in the widest possible sense – have on disease and health in general and on cancer in particular.

There are two things to say. Firstly, it does seem to be true that there is a range of factors that make people live longer, when we look at meta-analyses of large cohort studies. Following thousands of people over many years, it seems that in general, better income levels, education, less depression and so on, are associated with better health and less disease *of all sorts*. This may be via a range of intermediate factors which are likely to include taking up healthier lifestyles, using healthcare for prevention and so on. This does *not* mean, however, that any individual can say that they brought their cancer on themselves; in fact, given their particular physical disposition and exposures to risk factors, you may have delayed the onset of a cancer which was likely to happen in any case.

Secondly, there are other studies which appeared in the 1980s and 1990s to show that psychological interventions in patients with cancer had the effect of increasing survival. These studies have since been criticised and have not been replicated, though in bigger studies with more up-to-date study designs that allow for small differences in the illness itself and how it is expressed, therefore to be monitored. The general view at the moment is that while psychological interventions may help you engage with your treatment more effectively, by coping or tolerating it better, or by making you more likely to keep going with a treatment that you are undertaking, we don't have firm evidence that your mental approach, once diagnosed, will impact on your chances more than the treatment that you are having.

It is true that some very demanding treatments are more likely to be completed if you are in a reasonably good state beforehand – but these types of measures include how physically sturdy you are feeling, as well as emotionally.

In my work I am struck by how hard many of my patients are on themselves. They impose enormous burdens by demanding that they should 'be positive'. Often, friends and relatives will demand this too; even after the most difficult consultation they will emerge cheerfully focusing on only the good, or less bad, elements of what has been said. This may seem to be helpful; however, the person with the cancer is then doubly trapped; they have their own fears and anxieties – and they have nowhere to discuss them.

What is the role of psychology in cancer?

It can be as simple as knowing that in face of anxiety we stop taking in information and aren't going to remember much of what is said to us (the first experiments on this were done with WWII bomber pilots who ran out of fuel returning from bombing raids because, in their highly anxious state engendered by the raid, they weren't noticing that the fuel gauge was low). We also know that preparing patients for surgery and treatment by letting them know what to expect and how to get pain relief when they need it, makes recovery more speedy; we can manage anxiety and fear around investigations such as MRI, work with patients who have injection phobias, and offer self-management interventions like expressive writing, which has been shown to promote physical and mental recovery in surgery and cancer.

It can extend to making use of the research evidence that we have on how medical systems work, and how patients and their close ones function within them. How much does a patient remember when they come out of a doctor's appointment? Even at a straightforward GP appointment most people interviewed afterwards remember only 15 per cent of what is said. The doctor is convinced they conveyed the information. They said it: but it wasn't taken away by their patient.

And how much worse is it if the situation is more threatening? 'After I heard the word "cancer" I couldn't hear anything else.'

You may have to make life-changing decisions in a very small time frame; moving from hoping to have children to knowing that you never can; balancing decisions between treatments when you are offered information; what does it really mean to you to be told 15 per cent chance versus 20 per cent chance? Our patients are navigating a great deal of distress and loss, and we need to tread the right path between information over-load and under-load.

What can I do?

Simple self-help can include accepting all the help that is offered and being explicit with those in your world who say: 'What can I do to help?' (There is a very useful book by Deborah Hutton with this title, on how to manage the social world as a patient with cancer.)

Be explicit about things that can be accepted practically – some communities offer food, child care, accompanying to hospital. Volunteers are now wide-spread and these may be local, or you can find them via national organisations such as Macmillan who train their own volunteers.

Minimise your use of the internet. Try to make sure that you are getting information that really maps onto your own case, and this is usually best managed via your medical team and the sources that they advise you to access.

Don't feel that you have to tell everybody all the details of where your cancer story is, just because they asked. You are in new territory now, with different rules. You need to give yourself permission *not* to answer the question 'How are you?' truthfully or fully, if that is exhausting. Many people describe getting home after a tough day and spending all evening on the phone to a range of friends, re-hashing what is happening. Or worse – having had a relatively cancer-free day and fielding such a call and being taken back into all the hardest parts, while they were having a good day.

The aim of managing cancer psychologically is not to repudiate or pretend it isn't there, but to deal with it when necessary and to be able to put it in the background of your life at other times and have *your* life.

Many of my patients work out a form of words to use so that they aren't caught unawares by such questions and blurt out things that they really don't want to be talking about. In the old days we didn't discuss cancer; even now you wouldn't be expected to give all the details of your stomach upset on a daily basis to friends and colleagues, so why feel pushed to do the same with your cancer?

Phrases like 'What about you?' or 'Let's talk about anything other than my illness; or 'I've spoken to my psychologist and we've agreed that it's not good for me to keep going over this, so I'm very happy to talk to you about anything else . . . ' Some people have a blog, or a group e-mail to family and friends. Often a friend or relative will tend to field such calls and requests for information – but this can eventually be too much for them; they are likely to be going through their own issues and often get less support, so be a little wary of the costs of doing it this way.

Assistance from professional psychologists is now available at all points of the patient journey, some via psychologists, many via counsellors, Clinical Nurse Specialists or other workers. Outside the NHS they may be available from third-sector community resources with psychological input, such as Maggie's Centres.

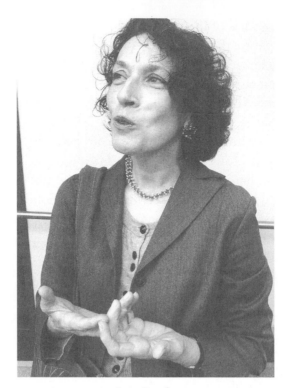

Sue Gessler

Conclusion

Is there one way to cope? No. There is a prescriptive quality today in many areas of our society, and the many texts available and beliefs expressed often have no space for individual differences. You are the person you were before your disease was diagnosed, and had your own particular approach to dealing with difficulties. To force you into an inauthentic copy of someone else's style is both dishonest and unhelpful. There are people for whom knowing what is the worst that could happen is containing. Others prefer their doctors to speak in more general terms and to hold within themselves uncertainties.

You will have your own journey – and your own process – and your own way of being through your journey may be very different from the one Gemma describes.

But it is yours.

Radiotherapy in the Treatment of Breast Cancer

DR SARAH HARRIS MRCP, FRCR
Clinical Oncologist – Radiotherapy

The reality of cancer is part of all our lives. We all know friends and family who have suffered and we can only marvel at their courage and determination, their resilience and their heroic acceptance of what they have to deal with. They set an example to us all.

DAME JOAN BAKEWELL DBE

Radiotherapy has evolved in the treatment of cancer over the last century. The modern radiotherapy machines operated by powerful computers and technology are a far cry from the low-energy machines used until a quarter of a century ago. These new machines offer highly targeted treatment maximising the beneficial effect while minimising the radiation dose to unwanted adjacent areas of the body, hence limiting the side effects

How Does Radiotherapy Work?

Beams of X-rays are generated from machines – the majority of which are called Linear Accelerators. As the X-rays pass through the body tissues, they cause changes in the chromosomes – the genetic material in the cells. The tissues of the normal body are able to repair these changes after each treatment but if there are any cancer cells in the area these are less efficient at the repair process and are likely to be killed.

After wide local excision (breast-conserving surgery) radiotherapy is delivered to the breast to reduce the chances of recurrence in the breast over the following ten years from up to 30 per cent to a much lower risk of 2–5 per cent. Some patients will also receive radiotherapy after a mastectomy – more likely if the patient has a large or node positive breast cancer.

Patients receiving radiotherapy after surgery are likely to have their course of treatment divided into 15–30 treatments called fractions. Each course of radiotherapy is personalised to the patient.

The Radiotherapy Team

Most patients will have met their Radiotherapy Consultant or deputy (also known as a Clinical Oncologist) at their outpatient consultation and have had the opportunity to discuss their proposed treatment and the possible benefits and side effects. Within the radiotherapy department the patient's main point of contact will be the radiotherapy technicians who operate the machines and in the UK are called Radiographers. These staff will work closely with the Consultant to provide expert treatment and care for the patient on a daily basis – getting to know the patient a little and reassuring them. They appreciate that it is often a very daunting time coming to the radiotherapy department, particularly for the first visit, and many patients are frightened. Breast care and specialist nurses also are likely to meet the patient during their radiotherapy course. Written information regarding the treatment is usually provided and many radiotherapy departments have information centres where patients can read further about their diagnosis and treatments in more detail with an experienced person to facilitate this.

Starting a Course of Radiotherapy

Modern radiotherapy is mapped out using 3-dimensional inform-ation from a CT scan (Computerised Tomography). Many patients will already have undergone a CT scan for diagnostic purposes but the radiotherapy planning scan is specific to the treatment. The patient lies on a couch identical to the couches on the treatment machines in a reproducible position usually with their arms above their head resting in supports. The CT scan is taken and then 2–3 small permanent marks are left on the skin around the breast area – these are the reference points for radiotherapy delivery each day of treatment.

There is often then a 1–2 week gap before starting radiotherapy. In this time the treatment beams and dose of radiotherapy are prescribed by the doctor. The dosimetry and physics staff then plan, calculate and most importantly check in several ways that the treatment to be delivered is correct.

As the treatment is delivered to a 2 mm accuracy, it is important that any swelling in the breast or chest wall area has settled before the CT scan is taken, as if the area continues to change shape the CT scan and planning process may need to be repeated.

Radiotherapy Delivery

Each day the patient attends for treatment at a specific appointment time. Most radiotherapy is delivered via a linear accelerator – a highly specialised machine which produces high-energy X-rays used for treatment rather than diagnostic purposes. The area to be treated – called the target volume – is the whole breast or the chest wall after mastectomy. The lymph gland area in the neck may also be treated if the patient has had significant involvement of the axillary lymph glands after surgery.

There are several technical terms detailing exactly how the radiotherapy is given:

Intensity Modulated Radiotherapy (IMRT) – used even in simple form in most breast cancer treatments. The shape and evenness of the beam are modified by small pieces of metal hidden in the head of the treatment machine to deliver a uniform dose of treatment throughout the breast area.

IGRT (Image Guided Radiotherapy) – most radiotherapy machines also have the ability to take simple X-ray or CT-like images during the treatment to verify that the treatment being delivered is the same as that planned.

Some patients will receive their radiotherapy from other machines – the commonest being the tomotherapy unit – which delivers both IMRT and IGRT. Cobalt machines were previously used in the UK but have largely been superseded by linear accelerators, except in less developed countries where they continue to provide reliable treatment and easy-to-maintain equipment.

A number of trials have been carried out to determine the number of treatments or fractions needed for each patient. In the UK most patients will receive 15 moderate-sized or 25 smaller treatments to the breast area each day – taking 3 or 5 weeks respectively. The

evidence suggests these two treatment regimes are similar in effect and side effects and many patients will receive the shortened course of treatment. Some patients will also receive 5–8 extra fractions as a 'boost' – an extra treatment concentrating on the tumour bed, the area where the tumour was removed from. This is most likely to be recommended in patients less than 50 years old with larger and grade 2 or 3 cancers. Patients who have undergone a mastectomy do not usually require the additional boost treatment.

Results and Side Effects

Radiotherapy is very successful in reducing the chances of recurrence around the breast, chest wall and lymph gland area to approximately 2 per cent at ten years and also may improve the chance of cure for some patients from their breast cancer.

The side effects of radiotherapy are feared by many patients – some of whom have horror stories from treatment delivered many years ago. Reassuringly for most patients, modern radiotherapy is a very safe treatment, given with very few and manageable side effects.

The immediate (also described as acute or early) side effects happen during the course of radiotherapy and for a few weeks after. The skin of the breast, chest wall or lymph gland area may become pink or red one or two weeks into treatment and areas of friction – under the breast and in the arm pit area – may become sore with superficial loss of the skin surface towards the end of the radio-therapy and for one or two weeks after. Creams and dressings would be suggested for comfort and the area heals shortly after treatment is complete.

The long-term side effects develop months or years after radio-therapy and for most patients are mild. The radiotherapy causes fibrosis or scar tissue to develop through the beam pathways causing the patient's breast to become firmer and occasionally change shape a little. The tissues underlying the breast may also be affected – often without causing symptoms. Approximately 1–2 cm of the front of the lung is treated – the scar tissue caused will not cause symptoms unless the patient's lung function was already compromised, for example by emphysema. With modern radiotherapy the heart is excluded from the radiotherapy field whenever possible. However, if a small part of the heart is treated the risk of heart disease more than ten years later rises by approximately 1 per cent. For most patients other risk factors for heart disease will be more relevant, such as raised blood pressure and cholesterol, diabetes, etc. Very rare effects of radiotherapy are an increased risk of developing another unrelated cancer or, if the lymph glands are treated, damage to the nerves to the arm.

Radiotherapy after Breast Reconstruction

Radiotherapy affects both implant and tissue flap reconstructions by causing damage to small blood vessels in the skin and underlying tissue, as well as the formation of scar tissue. The plastic surgeons would prefer radiotherapy to be avoided after reconstruction; however, for some patients it is advised, to reduce the chance of recurrence around the breast area. As a result of radiotherapy, a fibrotic hard capsule may form around an implant causing hardening and alteration of the shape of the implant. Some patients may have an expander inserted at the time of their mastectomy which stretches the skin and underlying tissue and this is replaced by an implant a few months after radiotherapy is complete. Scar tissue may form after a flap-based reconstruction causing hardening and shape change of the area. Reconstruction combined with radiotherapy is now common in the treatment of breast cancer and both areas have improved significantly in the last five years.

Future Radiotherapy Directions

The planning and delivery capabilities of radiotherapy equipment will continue to improve to allow further improvements in the delivery of the radiotherapy dose while sparing the surrounding tissues from the beams.

The deep inspiratory breath hold (DIBH) is a technique which is gaining in popularity for the treatment of some patients with left-sided breast cancers to reduce the radiotherapy dose delivered to the heart. For certain patients, if they took a moderate sized breath which they held for approximately 20 seconds, the heart would move away from the treatment area. The radiotherapy beam would only be activated when the patient was in this position – called respiratory gating. This technique would only be suitable for patients who were able to hold their breath for this time and where this technique would improve the radiotherapy dose delivered near the heart.

Intra-operative radiotherapy is gaining popularity. The patient may be given a dose of radiotherapy to the tumour bed at the time of surgical removal of the tumour. One such technique is the Intrabeam. Despite some concerns about the adequacy of such treatments, which treat only the breast area close to the original tumour, the TARGIT trial in 2010 reported good results without an increase in tumour recurrence in the early years of follow-up. Potentially this and other similar techniques offer a one-off treatment or a substitute for the tumour bed boost.

Palliative Radiotherapy

Non-curative radiotherapy is usually given for control of symptoms when the cancer has spread beyond the breast and is most commonly used for treatment of the bones. The treatment is usually given as a shorter course commonly by linear accelerators. New treatment machines giving precise small-field radiotherapy – stereotactic radiotherapy is gaining in numbers. The Cyberknife is such a machine which delivers high doses of radiotherapy to small areas. In time these techniques may be used for the treatment of early breast cancer.

Conclusion

Radiotherapy, along with drug treatments, has improved enormously in the past decade in terms of success and reduction in side effects. The combination of treatments has a bright future in the treatment of breast cancer.

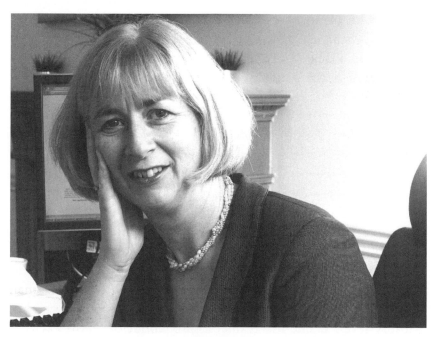

Sarah Harris

New Drugs

PROFESSOR PAUL ELLIS MD FRACP
PROFESSOR JUSTIN STEBBING FRCP, FRCPath, PhD

One day there will be a cure. Until then, I hope that this book will encourage everyone affected by cancer to never give up.

DAME JUDI DENCH CH DBE

Introduction

Over the past two decades, through a combination of detection at an earlier stage, and the development of better treatments, breast cancer survival has continued to improve. There are currently more than half a million women in the UK who are alive and well having been treated for breast cancer and four out of five women who present with breast cancer remain alive and well five years later. However, each year, 1 to 2 per cent of previously treated women will develop a treatable relapse and approximately a third of these women will develop metastases and subsequently die of their disease. One of the best ways to try and further improve the survival of breast cancer patients is by developing newer more effective drug therapies. The last decade has seen a revolution in our understanding of the molecular workings of the cancer cell, and with this has come the identification of therapeutic targets within the cell against which new cancer drugs can be developed.

In the last few years, we have understood that a disease such as breast cancer is not just one disease, but it may in fact be hundreds of different diseases with considerable histologic and functional heterogeneity. New drugs being developed now take this into account and as we closely link the clinic to the laboratory and vice versa, there is an understanding that real change is occurring at every level. If one asked oncologists about the most exciting developments, most would focus on the era of new drugs and personalised therapy, that is, giving the right treatment to the right tumour at the right time. Key to this is the fact that it isn't just one treatment that makes a difference, but improvements in a combination of therapies including surgery, radiotherapy, as well as hormonal therapy targeting receptors in the cytoplasm of growing cells, chemotherapy that attacks the DNA and its machinery in the nucleus, and the new biologic agents such as the monoclonal antibodies (for example trastuzumab) and tyrosine kinase inhibitors (for example lapatinib) or bevacizumab that target cell growth factor receptors. What is even more exciting is that there are now next generation drugs building on these advances, such as new treatments that can actually link chemotherapy to antibody therapy in one single molecule, to attack the cancer much more precisely with fewer side effects or toxicities.

Starting with basic science work and an understanding of what drives the different types of breast cancer, the flow of research data concerning the basis of breast cancer is rapidly increasing in speed and complexity. In response, many projects are seeking to ensure that there are appropriate informatics tools, systems and databases available to manage and exploit this flood of information, especially as we enter a genomics era in which sequences of different tumours arenow being used as well as novel biomarkers that can be used to select the right therapy. New systems are being set up for auto-mated management of data flows, quality control in the laboratory and clinic and, most importantly, making sure we understand our patients. Along with emerging drugs and technologies that enhance both quantity and quality of life, collaborative advances should help to create a powerful environment for 'beating breast cancer'.

The Biology of Breast Cancer

Amongst the different types of breast cancer there are three major groupings that are clinically relevant: oestrogen receptor positive disease; HER2 positive disease; and triple negative disease – named in response to the three main receptors (the two hormone receptors – oestrogen and progesterone receptor, and HER2) on the surface of breast cancer cells. Hormonal therapies, including drugs such as tamoxifen, that blocks the oestrogen receptor, aromatase inhibitors such as Anastrozole, Letrozole or exemestane, that prevent estrogen production and Fulvestrant that degrades the receptor, are used across the world to stop the signals into the nucleus of cancer cells from the oestrogen receptor. Trastuzumab (Herceptin) binds to the HER2 receptor on the cell surface and blocks that, and this has been one of the most revolutionary anti-cancer drugs, demonstrating significant improvements in survival for patients with this type of breast cancer. Oncologists, pathologists and geneticists have also used the term triple negative breast cancer since 2006, referring to an absence of these particular receptors in 15–20 per cent of cases. The use of lots of names, however, just reflects our own uncertainty as to the true nature of this disease, unlike oestrogen receptor positive disease (70 per cent) or HER2 positive disease (20 per cent). One can have oestrogen receptor positive and HER2 positive disease that benefits from hormonal therapy and Trastuzumab, but the only treatment for triple negative disease up till recently has been cytotoxic chemotherapy. The question of whether there is a specific, identifiable cell in the normal breast from which any breast cancers arise is controversial and considerable research is focusing on this. All types of breast cancer can ultimately relapse although the relapse rates can differ and patterns of relapse can differ too. For example, hormone receptor positive disease can relapse in the bones after many years whereas triple negative disease can produce widespread metastases quickly. HER2 positive disease has a propensity for the central nervous system but many of all of these types are cured when the breast cancer presents at an early stage.

Conventional chemotherapies are initially effective in controlling tumour growth in many breast cancers, yet many patients relapse over time. At least two major explanations exist for these observations. The first is that all cancer cells become resistant to the drugs resulting in decreased overall sensitivity to therapy over time. In this case, the relative proportion of cells in residual tumours with tumourigenic properties would be expected to be similar before and after treatment. The second explanation is that a rare subpopulation of cells with tumourigenic potential is resistant to therapy right from the beginning of treatment. In this case, the relative proportion of cells in residual tumours with tumourigenic properties would be expected to increase after treatment. Analogous to the propensity of dandelion roots to regenerate weeds, regrowth of tumours from an intrinsically chemotherapy-resistant sub-population has been termed the 'dandelion hypothesis'. Consistent with this hypothesis, it has previously been shown that the gene expression pattern of residual tumour cells surviving after treatment is different from that of cells in the initial tumour, with differential expression of genes involved in cell cycle arrest and survival pathways in particular. This hypothesis provides a unified explanation for the successes and failures of chemotherapy: namely, that although the majority of cells in the original tumour may be killed by chemotherapy, the most important target, a small population of therapy-resistant cancer cells that possess tumourigenic capacity, is spared, thereby allowing tumour regrowth. These cells are thought to be cancer stem cells, which possess very unusual properties. A combination of treatments that target both subpopulations is therefore critical to prevent tumour regrowth and relapse.

Clinical development

Cancer drug trials have typically involved a traditional evidence-based approach that focuses on treating patient populations with molecularly uncharacterised disease, culminating in large, pivotal, randomised therapeutic trials aimed at regulatory approval. Usually, such an approach aims to improve survival or a surrogate of survival by at best a few months and a good example of these are all the trials in metastatic breast cancer. Here, there has been increased regulatory scrutiny in breast cancer studies in which the end points and design of the trials are now being looked at very closely to make sure the effects of these drugs are real and meaningful for patients. Sometimes this is referred to as showing the drugs are 'clinically significant' not just 'statistically significant' (that is, they work in real people not just on paper). There are growing concerns with the previous 'one size fits all' approach, as demonstrated by the high proportion of negative large randomised studies and / or the limited benefits observed in the minority that actually are positive. Moreover, these trials define the best therapy for the average patient, whereas they may not be optimal for the individual with a particular biological subtype of cancer. Large numbers of patients have been entered into these trials in an attempt to minimise the effects of heterogeneity, both with respect to patients and the type of cancer, and to widen the proportion of individuals suitable for a particular drug.

The first signs of change are that the degree of benefit from a new treatment is now being recognised in early clinical trials, before large ones are pursued. The attrition rate in pharmaceutical, bio-technology and investigator-led academic studies is increasing, so drugs that don't work are not being 'flogged' to show that they might. Currently, most new drug approvals are for agents directed against existing targets such as the cell surface receptors in breast cancer that drive blood vessel growth (the vascular endothelial growth factor receptor, VEGFR) with only a minority being novel. This seems less likely to be due to the lack of suitable targets but rather due to the difficulty, time required, cost and attrition rate in development, as well as lack of proper validation of novel targets. The critical first step, if the process is to succeed, is a strong biologic basis for the target. Necessary, but not sufficient, is the identific-ation of an altered molecular target in the cancer (or any disease) to provide a therapeutic window and therefore a clear basis for selective cytotoxicity (cell death) with absolute or relative sparing of normal cells. Inherent within this is the definition of a target patient population and a practical method to identify them (for example, a biomarker or other diagnostic). Successful examples of this approach would include the PARP inhibitors in triple negative breast cancer, although laboratory success does not always translate into clinical success.

Laboratory Development

There does seem to be an understanding now that we need to identify targets that cancer cells are absolutely reliant on so that when their functions are blocked, the cells die. Preferably, these will be targets to which resistance is not easily gained. However, we do not yet seem to recognise that our understanding of how a cancer cell is wired versus normal cells is at best rudimentary. What one calls discrete pathways are complex interacting networks and thus inhibiting one step may have unpredictable consequences because of, for example, negative feedback loops or positive reinforcement. All of these pathways are linked, and changing one aspect can change many others, sometimes not for the greater good.

Systems-based computationally intensive approaches that account for some of these issues are now being used, for the first time, but they are in their infancy. Along with this, animal models that mimic the clinical disease are better, such as orthotopic or natural transplantation as opposed to xenografts from a different animal. It also seems likely that the cost of the newer agents will mandate the requirement for a highly selective patient group to which these drugs can be given.

Considering the three umbrella types of breast cancer in further detail, it is worthwhile discussing some of the progress being made.

1   *Triple Negative Disease*

This umbrella term can also be used to include rarer genetic breast cancers, such as those arising in women who have mutations in their BRCA1 or BRCA2 genes. Most mutations in cancer are not passed down to one's children, but these mutations are hereditary. In cells that carry BRCA1 and BRCA2 mutations, one of the two major DNA repair methods, known as homologous recombination, is non-functional. However, the other major repair method, known as base-excision repair, compensates for that loss. PARP-1 is an enzyme involved in DNA repair, especially in the repair of tumour cells. Thus, the PARP-1 enzyme is a target that, once hit and inhibited, leads to cell death and this has been called 'synthetic lethality'. It is thought that some types of sporadic triple negative breast cancer also have functional impairment of the BRCA pathway even though they don't have an obvious mutation evident. It is felt that they may also benefit from drugs such as the PARP inhibitors although research is ongoing in an attempt to prove this. There are almost certainly other tumours with defects in homologous recombination that should make them targets for PARP inhibition therapy too, but much more work is needed here.

2   *Hormone Receptor Positive Disease*

Although oestrogen receptor positive disease that relapses can be treated with different methods of anti-estrogenic therapy, usually at some point the illness becomes endocrine or hormone resistant, and other forms of therapy are required. For example, when it has spread to the bones, bisphosphonates or the new RANK-ligand inhibitors can be used to selectively target that disease. But for the most part there is no standard in this setting, and patient factors and the pattern of disease determine treatment as opposed to the gene expression of the cancer. Underpinning this, there is no standard model to explain endocrine resistance or, more importantly, study it in the laboratory. It used to be thought that patients lost their oestrogen receptor or it might become mutated, but now we know this doesn't occur. What seems to happen is a complex cascade of events that leads to the adding of a biochemical phosphate group to the receptor. When this occurs, it can still move to the nucleus and turn on breast cancer and cell division genes. We now know that a newly discovered protein in the cytoplasm can turn on the oestrogen receptor. Remarkably, this protein is new to humans and may explain too why humans are the only animals who frequently develop oestrogen receptor positive disease. Because of this, scientists are looking to make the 3-dimensional crystal structure of LMTK3, and then design key-shaped drugs to fit into its lock and block its activity.

3   *HER-2 Positive Disease*

The survival benefits with Trastuzumab have been staggering and it is free of chemotherapy-type side effects such as alopecia, infection and fatigue. Because we understand the target here, follow-on molecules have been made including Lapatinib which binds to the inner portion of the receptor, rather than the outer portion. Using Trastuzumab and Lapatinib together has been very interesting with high response rates but more exciting than this are the newer compounds, including those that have types of chemotherapy linked to the Trastuzumab itself. These are likely to be very effective but like the PARP inhibitors, the trials have been difficult to 'get right'. The most fascinating aspect of this is that if chemotherapy can be linked to an antibody like Trastuzumab, maybe it can linked to other antibodies too such as bevacizumab that targets blood vessel growth. Blood vessels deliver nutrients and oxygen to the body but also to cancers. Our understanding of blood vessel growth, so-called angiogenesis, is now much greater and thousands of patients benefit from inhibition of this process. Recent studies have now shown new molecular targets and basic principles, providing avenues for improving the therapeutic benefit from anti-angiogenic drugs. Examples of this include the VEGF, TGF-b, FGF superfamily, ANT and TIE signalling systems, the NOTCH and WNT signalling systems, integrins and proteases, junctional molecules, chemokines, G-protein coupled receptors and tyroskine kinase inhibitors (TKIs).

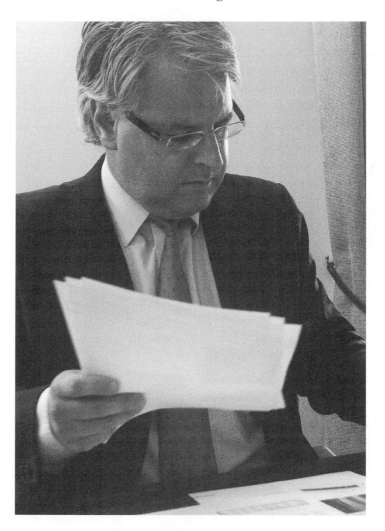

Paul Ellis

Conclusions

In the short term use of current drugs should be optimised and a further step forward would be the discovery of predictive bio-markers to identify patients who are much more likely to respond to treatment. Thus far, only a few candidates for predictive bio-markers have been identified, and they emerged from small studies that require prospective validation in larger randomised studies. It is likely, however, that the major advances in further improving breast cancer survival will come from optimising the use of the newer targeted therapies and understanding which biological sub-types of breast cancer benefit from which treatments. For example, little is understood about the mechanisms of growth of tiny lesions, so-called micrometastases that we cannot see using our scanning equipment, and understanding the mechanistic differences between drugs that need chemotherapy with them to work (for example, anti-VEGFR antibodies) and those that don't (for example, tyrosine kinase inhibitors) will be critical to formulate design of the most effective anticancer treatments. Collaboration and taking risks with drug development will also be critical.

These are exciting times in cancer, led by an inflection in our understanding of what makes cancer cells grow, driven in part by an explosion of our knowledge of genomics. A tight integration between preclinical and clinical research will be needed to achieve our goals.

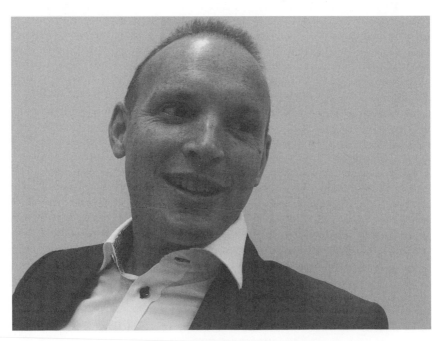

Justin Stebbing

Living Well

DR MICHELLE KOHN MB, BS BSc MRCP

Director of the Living Well Programme at LOC

When I was a child cancer was referred to as the Big C . . . the disease that dared not be named. Prognosis usually promised fatality. Today, it's a measure of progress that we refer to its full name. It is also now common for people to survive it. Possibly in my children's adulthood cancer will be regarded with the same equanimity as all those diseases that, in another century, meant death but now as an interruption of life, not the end of it.

HELENA BONHAM CARTER CBE

Cancer treatment, and its aftermath, can feel immensely disempowering. Many patients ask me, 'How can I take some control over what is happening to me?' or 'How can I get my life back?' Living Well addresses these questions. We are the safe, credible, supportive pair of hands that guides you through the emotional and practical minefield of treatment – and beyond.

I joined LOC, Leaders in Oncology Care, in 2009 to set up a programme for people whose cancer treatment had finished. Our founding oncologists rightly recognised that when treatment ends, patients often feel abandoned. They might be facing all sorts of ongoing physical and emotional challenges, but suddenly they are on their own, and they ask, 'Is that it?' Living Well was set up to offer care beyond medical treatment – a much-needed resource. Little did I know, then, how far and fast it would grow. I am now part of a programme that represents the future of cancer care – and it is a huge privilege.

A cancer diagnosis brings enormous psychological and emotional challenges. People often feel frightened, vulnerable, angry or low, both during and after treatment. Cancer can disrupt relationships, family life, body image, or career. All this has a huge impact on quality of life. Yet these issues are, too often, overlooked by a medical establishment that is focused on clinical treatment and outcomes.

The core of Living Well is a programme of six weekly classes, held in a supportive group setting. In essence, we empower people – whether they have just been diagnosed or have finished treatment – with information, understanding, camaraderie and key coping skills.

To do this, we have an amazing team of clinical specialists and experts from a range of disciplines. Some come from oncology: we have over forty oncologists from the major London cancer centres as well as our own team of renowned in-house doctors. Others are from the broader field of wellbeing: we have specialist nurses, psychologists, nutritionists and exercise experts, relaxation and beauty 'gurus'. We are also developing strong links with doctors who have an interest in the effects of cancer and its treatment – for instance, specialists working with bone health, clinical genetics or fertility. Together, we help people not just to live with and after cancer, but to thrive.

The absolute key to Living Well is the group environment. Meeting weekly, about twenty patients quickly realise that they are not alone. There is a lot of laughter – and a few tears too – but no pressure to perform or 'share'. The relief people feel when they realise that it isn't mad to lie awake at night worrying, it isn't weak or silly to feel low, and it isn't self-indulgent to care about how you feel (or look) is immense. In fact, one of the most motivating parts of my role is seeing how the programme transforms people – even those who initially came through the door feeling sceptical or uncertain.

There is more to all this than camaraderie, though. As a doctor, I have seen how overwhelming the effects of cancer and its treatment can be, both physically and mentally. Your body may be facing numerous challenges, such as overwhelming fatigue, 'chemo-brain' symptoms, neuropathy or weight changes. And your emotions can be all over the place. Our weekly sessions teach patients key skills to cope with these, and other, challenges.

One session, for instance, is devoted to exercise, something that is increasingly recognised to be very important to cancer out-comes, both during and after treatment. Our exercise experts offer individually tailored ways to become active and fit, tackling issues such as fatigue and pain and motivation. Our dieticians, meanwhile, show patients how to eat for maximum health. The emphasis is not just on nutrition, but on the joy of good food, a pleasure that is too often lost during treatment. Our sessions end with a delicious, chef-cooked meal, which is always uplifting.

Our in-house psychologist provides people with simple tools to cope with emotional and physical challenges. You might, for instance, learn a simple breathing method that keeps you calm when going for a scan. Or you might learn ways to cope with fatigue, building up your levels of activity gradually, rewarding yourself each step of the way. These techniques are all evidence-based, and really do make a difference to quality of life, whatever kind of cancer you have, and whatever stage you are at. You can't possibly live well, if you are struggling with unmanageable feelings or symptoms.

We also offer sensible, practical advice on anything from getting back to work, to long-term medical plans. In addition to the six-week programme itself, we have stand-alone workshops and clinics to tackle specific issues. There are, for instance, sessions for carers (family members and loved ones), who are often overlooked and yet desperately need help and advice too. And there are clinics on sexual wellbeing, from our doctor who specialises in psychosexual medicine.

Cancer can be an isolating, frightening experience. To share your fears and confusion with people who really understand what you are going through is invaluable. I love the fact that people tend to stay in touch after the programme finishes; we are even talking about creating a 'Friends of Living Well' group to extend this sense of community and support.

Still, it is not just the human side of Living Well that matters to me. Its clinical effectiveness is vital. As a doctor, I am fascinated by integrated and supportive cancer care. There is increasing scientific evidence that quality of life can have a direct impact on cancer outcomes. This is why I passionately believe that Living Well is not an 'add-on' to cancer care. It is a central component of it.

Since our launch, we have expanded to pre-empt and prevent many of the challenges patients face, from diagnosis onwards. None of this is a luxury, or a 'touchy-feely' extra. It has huge clinical relevance in oncology today. Increasingly, cancer is becoming a chronic illness that can be managed with medications. We do not just want people to survive longer, but to thrive. I have been Medical Advisor to Macmillan Cancer Support, and to Breakthrough Breast Cancer. I have also worked with organisations in the USA, where 'survivorship' programmes, and integrative oncology are very advanced. I truly believe that Living Well is the future of cancer care.

We have been asked to expand, and there is enormous interest from within the NHS, as oncologists recognise that these are vital aspects of treatment and recovery. We are creating a sustainable model that, I hope, will become part of standard cancer treatment. Helping to orchestrate this sea-change is an immense privilege. Our medical experts say that they learn as much – if not more – from Living Well patients as the patients learn from them. This is why the programme is so exciting for me. Quite simply, it changes lives.

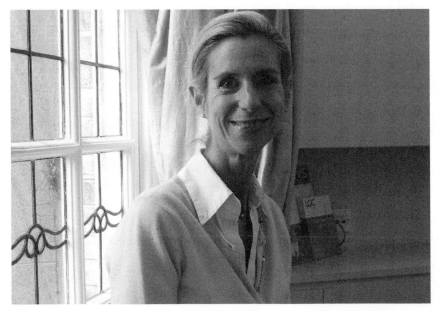

Michelle Kohn

Look Good . . . Feel Better: 1

Unveiling Inner Beauty and Promoting Self-confidence with the Healing Power of Lipstick

MARGARET HEWSON

Director of Look Good . . . Feel Better, South Africa

Who said a little lipstick can't make you feel better – someone who has never felt so emotionally low that she doesn't want to leave the protective walls of her own bedroom. And this is how many women facing cancer feel.

It is as a result of the power of lipstick that my story unfolds . . .

In 1987, a physician asked former Personal Care Products Council President Ed Kavanaugh how he could organise a 'makeover' for a woman in cancer treatment who was experiencing dramatic appearance side effects. The woman was so depressed and self-conscious she would not venture outside her hospital room. Kavanaugh made some calls and was able to provide cosmetics and a cosmetologist – and the makeover transformed not only the woman's look, but also her outlook. She felt happier and less burdened, and laughed for the first time in weeks.

With such a profound result, the Personal Care Products Council recognised the opportunity for its industry to help more women maintain their confidence and self-esteem. The programme – dubbed *Look Good . . . Feel Better* – launched with two group workshops at Memorial Sloan-Kettering Cancer Center in New York and Georgetown University's Lombardi Cancer Center in Washington, DC, in 1989. Today there are 23 independent licensed international *Look Good . . . Feel Better* affiliate programmes across the globe.

How privileged I am to have been involved in the launch of the LGFB Foundation in South Africa in 2004. Born and bred in Africa and having taught senior school children for many years I was more than ready to spread my wings and take on a new challenge. My friend Marie, who had been exposed to the LGFB programme in Paris, returned to Johannesburg fired up to bring the amazing gift of the LGFB programme to South African women with cancer. Her enthusiasm was contagious and in 2004 under the auspices of the Cosmetic, Toiletry and Fragrance Association South Africa, *Look Good . . . Feel Better* South Africa was born.

As Programme Director I have had the incredible joy of knowing that well over 13,000 SA women have benefited from a LGFB workshop in a very special way, and it has often been a turning point in their cancer journey . . . so allow me to introduce you in a more personal way to a LGFB workshop.

It's 9.30 a.m. and the team of well-trained LGFB volunteers arrive at the oncology unit, walk through to a large airy room laden with bags of cosmetic products required for the 12-step skin care and make-up regime. At 10.00 women begin to arrive, often looking apprehensive and vulnerable. After a warm introduction the workshop begins and those wearing wigs are invited to remove them should they wish. Hesitantly wigs are whisked off heads, the last promise of a woman's crowning glory. But all is not lost and smiles return when the amazing contents of the cosmetic bag given to each lady are revealed.

It's now time for the beauty professional to guide the twelve ladies through each step, addressing the appearance-related side effects that they may be experiencing as a result of their chemo and radiation therapy, which can be devastating – loss of hair, brows, and lashes and changes to the skin to name a few, commonly occur. These changes can undermine self-esteem and make coping with the disease much more difficult. The journey is different for everyone but there is a common thread of vulnerability, fear, uncertainly and loss of control.

As the workshop continues the ladies visibly relax and have fun learning new techniques to help them to address their appearance-related side effects as they experiment with new colours and apply their make-up, assisted by caring, supportive LGFB volunteers who are humbled as they observe the ladies looking at their reflection with new-found hope and confidence.

How often there is someone sitting around the table whose hair has recently re-grown and now can sincerely encourage another fearful that hers is about to fall out. Exploring new ideas with hats, turbans and wigs is always enthusiastically received.

It is truly wonderful to witness these women's spirits literally rise before our eyes and their confidence and self-esteem restored. There is a sparkle back in their eyes, an excitement in their voices and an inner confidence that 'No matter what is happening to me, I will get through it, and I am not alone.'

It is hard to find words to express the value of the social inter-action of the ladies as they enjoy tea afterwards; share their stories and exchange contact details. They have found a new friend, someone who really understands. Together they leave the sessions laughing, looking fantastic and ready to deal with their disease and face the world again.

In South Africa these complimentary, product – neutral, non-medical workshops are offered to patients in public and private oncology units. Many women, especially those from rural areas, have never worn make-up before or even owned a lipstick. The diversity of languages spoken here makes it necessary to offer the workshop material in English, Afrikaans, Sotho, Zulu and Xhosa.

The importance of knowing you are not alone when faced with a life-threatening disease that challenges the very essence of your femininity is immeasurable. Yes, your support group surrounds you, your family, friends and medical professionals but sometimes what you really want is to do is spend a few hours with women who are on a similar journey – to share stories and laughter in a warm and welcoming environment that makes you feel you're still engaged in the joy of living and this is where we at *Look Good . . . Feel Better* are able to help.

We also offer special workshops for men and teenage cancer patients.

None of this would be possible firstly without the incredible support from the cosmetic industry providing finances and pro-ducts, and secondly the hundreds of volunteers who generously give of their time, energy and expertise to support these courageous woman. Proudly LGFB is the bridge between patients, brands, volunteers, hospitals, oncologists and the healing process.

Sadly the number of women diagnosed with cancer each year

shows little sign of decreasing but on a positive note, with new treatments, many more women are winning their journey with cancer.

Globally the LGFB programme receives extensive recognition and support from healthcare professionals involved in patient care and treatment, who bear testimony to the basic thinking behind it – if you look good you feel better.

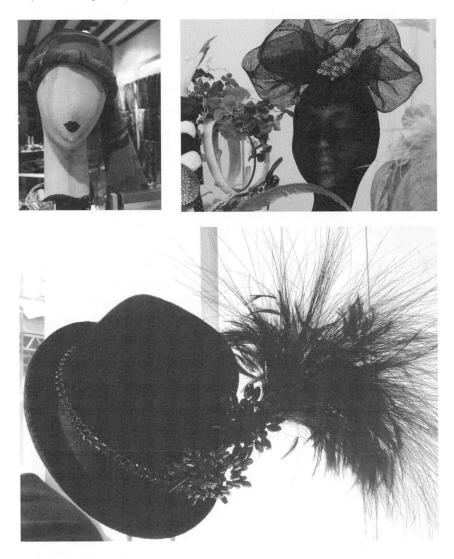

Look Good . . . Feel Better: 2

SARAHJANE ROBERTSON

Executive Director of Look Good . . . Feel Better, UK

'Look Good . . . Feel Better' – the name says it all – and for over twenty years that's what the 'team' at LGFB have been striving for in order to bring a little normality and control back into women's lives whilst they are battling through their cancer treatment.

I was fortunate to have been introduced to LGFB ten years ago and I have to admit to being a bit sceptical about how skincare and make-up workshops could actually help a woman when she clearly had so many other life-changing issues to cope with. Once I'd experienced my first session in London I was hooked – the difference that two hours made to twelve women was astounding and I've been working for *Look Good . . . Feel Better* in the UK ever since.

My wonderful colleague and friend, Margaret, in South Africa has explained how women react to our workshops and I'd like to highlight what it takes to actually pull it all together.

LGFB started in the USA over twenty years ago and quickly spread to Canada, Australia, New Zealand and the UK so we are the 'oldest' of our 24-strong team of countries. Between us we have supported over 1,000,000 women and our individual programmes continue to grow and develop alongside helping new countries just starting to get involved. We are able to share expertise and experience in all vital areas such as structure, fundraising, staffing, hospital liaison, volunteer recruitment, product support and all other aspects of running a national charity.

Spending time with the women we support is what makes our roles incredibly rewarding and worthwhile. Most of us come from commercial backgrounds and to be in a role that touches people's lives in such a positive and effective way is something we all truly value.

There are very many organisations and individuals who all pull

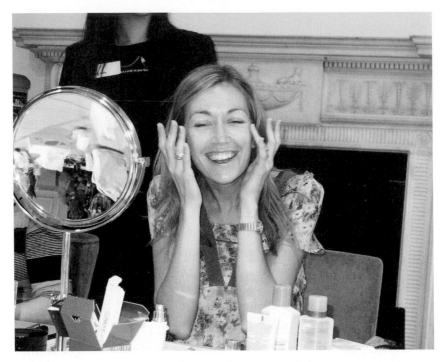

Look Good . . . Feel Better workshop

together as a 'team' to make LGFB possible around the world, and foremost amongst these is the entire beauty industry. I can't think of another industry where hundreds of companies and brands – all working in a highly competitive marketplace – put aside their professional rivalries and pool their support behind a charity they help to make possible. In the UK alone we have over 35 member companies and brands working alongside us, supporting us with volunteer beauty consultants, extensive product donations for our patient gift bags, expertise at board level and sponsorship, promotional and fundraising initiatives.

I can't possibly begin to really understand how another woman must feel when she is going through some of these dreadful treatments and I am humbled and inspired every time I visit a workshop and see how they just want to be treated as 'normal' and be able to go about their lives looking like 'themselves', not like the cancer patient they've been forced to become.

One of the things that always bubbles up at our workshops is the fabulous sense of humour of these brilliant ladies. Only last week someone said to me: 'It's awful losing all your hair like this.' I tried to empathise with this lady but she butted in with a big smile and said: '. . . yes, but I've saved a fortune on waxing,' which set all the other ladies off laughing.

That moment epitomises our sessions – women wanting to make each other laugh, wanting to share stories and let others who may be earlier in their treatment know that it will all be OK. They often swop 'phone numbers and people in their early twenties might make friends with someone in their fifties or sixties – they are all in the same boat and the confidence and strength imparted through our workshops lasts for many months to come.

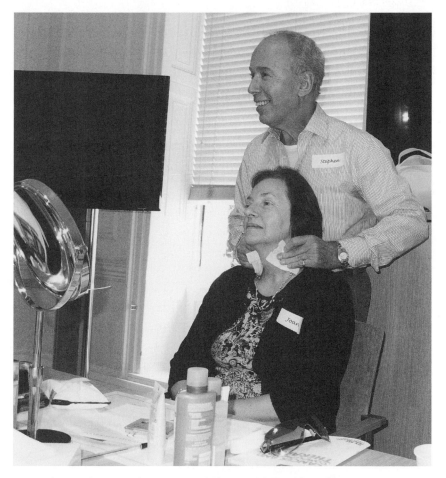

Look Good . . . Feel Better workshop with Stephen Glass, Face Facts
regional co-ordinator and a volunteer

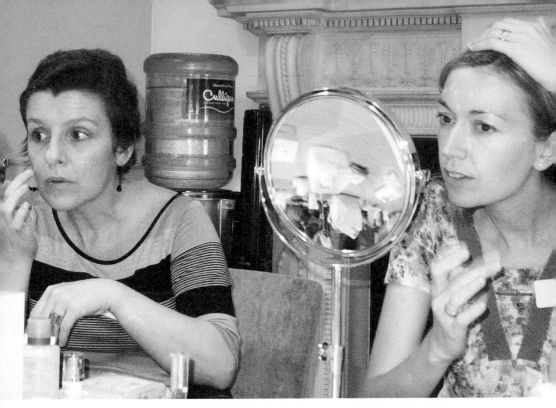

Look Good . . . Feel Better workshop

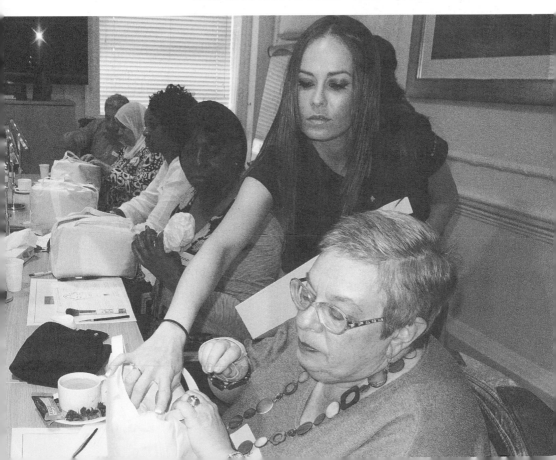

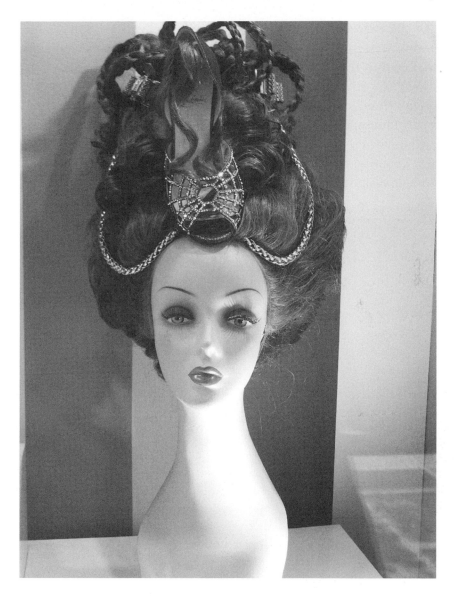

It's now over seventeen years since we launched LGFB in the UK and we currently run our sessions in 63 locations from the north of Scotland to the Channel Islands. Our key objective is to have the ability to reach out to every woman diagnosed with cancer in the country and currently we support over 11,000 face to face and many thousands more through our self-help materials and website.

Our motto is 'Let us put a smile on your face' and that's what we will continue to do for women living with cancer both in the UK and alongside all my LGFB friends and colleagues worldwide.

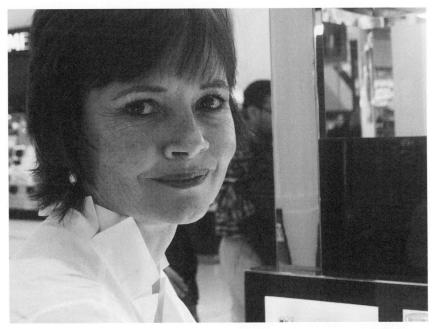

Sarahjane Robertson

Diet

JANE CLARKE BSc (Hons) SRD

Dietitian, cordon bleu chef and food writer

*There is not much of an upside to cancer, but the close brush with
the Grim Reaper does stimulate a re-think of priorities: suddenly it
is possible to stop working so hard, and give time to what matters:
family, friends, reflection, nature, music, books, whatever.*

PRUE LEITH CBE

I truly believe that timing is everything. Things are meant to
happen, when they happen, and for a woman who thrives on the
challenges of being an entrepreneur in my field, my world of food
and nourishment, meeting Gemma just before this manuscript was
put to bed proves this point beautifully. It was a chance query about
a side effect which had annoyingly lingered since Gemma finished
her treatment for breast cancer that led to us sitting down and
talking about how best she could nourish herself and find the body
she so keenly wanted to rediscover.

In Britain, despite there being some very sound scientific research
into how specific foods and ingredients can affect the immune
system and ultimately play some part in influencing the efficacy of
cancer treatments and how you ride the waves cancer throws at
your body, if you mention the words nutrition and diet to many
people, be this the wonderful doctors who support patients with
surgical or non-surgical cancer treatments, or other people going
through the cancer journey who are perhaps fed up with friends
and relatives bombarding them with albeit well-intentioned articles
from the internet, books or anecdotes, people tend to fall into one
of two camps. Either they say they don't want to start doing anything about the food they're eating, especially anything faddy or
extreme, when they're already having to deal with side effects and
all that a cancer diagnosis brings with it, or they become so worried

about the scary headline stories about, for example, dairy, meat and sugar being the devil's food, that food and eating become medicinal and worrisome.

As Gemma and I spend time together chatting about food, I see a huge part of my role, as a nutritionist (and clinical dietitian, but I rather like to leave those albeit professional-status-giving words to one side, as they just imply that I put the people I support on diets, which is far from the case) and a Cordon Bleu chef (which over the years defines me and the different way I treat the people who come to me), simply as being able to inspire and titillate the imagination and give people delicious ideas as to how our bodies can incorporate nourishing ingredients into our lifestyles. When you're going through the cancer journey, not only is there the necessity to push through the anxious times, when the last thing you feel like doing is to eat, yet your body so needs the nourishment to give you strength and the brain power to make the right decisions, but also, as you go through treatment, you need to get around its side effects – nausea, fatigue, bloating, swallowing difficulties, feeling low emotionally, etc. One of the most troublesome of these to women who go through breast cancer treatment is weight gain – as if having the disease wasn't enough, being left with a body which doesn't even feel like you. So often hormonal treatments can cause weight gain and / or menopausal symptoms, and while food can't provide any miracle solutions, tweaking the way you eat, the ingredients you choose, how you put them together and use them at different times of the day, can help you find the body you want to see when you look in the mirror. For instance, if you find that bread causes you to feel bloated, you could either try something like a spelt bread (spelt being an ancestor of the traditional wheat, and although it still contains gluten, many find that it seems easier to digest), or juggle with the time of day at which you eat it – it could be that it sits better during the evening than in the middle of the day, when traditionally so many people grab a sandwich and then feel lousy afterwards.

This wonderful book is not the place to dwell on getting too bogged down in the science of nutrients, but great words to look out for include antioxidants (more about these in a moment), choosing good as opposed to bad fats (generally the trans fats, and also it's not ideal to have too much saturated animal fat, such as butter, cream, etc.) and using them mindfully. Drizzle a delicious olive oil over a salad full of all sorts of colourful ingredients (this is one of the tricks of the trade, to choose food with your eyes, for it's the varying colours of vegetables, be this Chantenay carrots, Romano peppers, watercress, deep red cherry tomatoes, roasted young beetroot or courgettes and English peas, and the fact that they're vegetables and fruits that makes them one of our best sources of antioxidants such as vitamin C and beta-carotene, which help our body fight free radicals, the damaging substances our cells hate), or quickly pan-fry a piece of responsibly sourced salmon in a little cold-pressed rapeseed oil, which has one of the best fat profiles, being rich in the beneficial omega-3 fatty acids, and serve it with some steamed new potatoes and a warm chickpea, fresh mint, avocado and shallot salad.

I love to talk about breakfasts, which can be so much more than a bowl of cereal (whose labels are so often confusing) – I'm getting known as the Bramley apple woman, because one of the breakfasts I not only love myself, being lucky enough to live surrounded by ancient apple trees, so that having a plentiful supply is the under-statement, is stewed apple, which I tend to make at the weekend, in a big pot, which I then keep in the fridge and delve into each morning to provide an apple base (gorgeous chilled or, on colder mornings, warmed up to make a warm apple purée), to which I add a selection and variety of other fruits, such as blackberries, rasp-berries, sliced figs (fresh or dried), and then top with some thick Greek-style natural yoghurt, toasted walnuts and a drizzle of honey. Yes, I use yoghurt, and I try to reassure anyone who has come across the scary headlines about dairy being bad for people with cancer that there isn't anything sound in these stories – it's fine for us to include some dairy in our diet, and indeed there is some research to show that foods rich in calcium can help encourage the production of cancer-protective substances in the bowel, which get absorbed into the body. If you're worried about the fat content of dairy foods, go for either a semi-skimmed or a 1 per cent fat milk (both which contain just as much calcium as full cream and can feel lighter on the digestion and are less calorie-heavy too), and if you're a cheese lover, as I am, use a mature cheese, something like an aged

Comte, Gruyère, Pecorino or Parmesan, or of course one of our wonderful British Cheddars such as Keen's or Montgomery. Use a cheese slicer and shave off thin slices – this gives you a melt-in-your-mouth cheese hit, which with the high surface area of the shavings (as opposed to grabbing a chunk of cheese), satiates – how I love the word satiety, true satisfaction from eating.

The point of satiety is an important one when we're talking about losing some unwanted weight post cancer treatment, or indeed not gaining too much weight while you're undergoing active therapy, as so often the drugs (such as steroids or hormonal therapies) either increase our hunger or seem to stop us feeling full and satiated as efficiently and as soon as we used to, so if we're not careful the weight can creep on. As well as the types of foods we eat, the way we eat has an impact here, and this is where I get a piece of paper out and illustrate the way our mouth, jaw, stomach, all communicate with the satiety centre in the brain. Imagine that there are, say, eight little light bulbs in the satiety centre which all need to light up before we feel full – eating slowly, chewing so that the jaw can send signals back to light up some of the bulbs, savouring our food, that is, concentrating as we eat all those wonderful flavours, and – another thing which really seems to work – juggling different textures and tastes within a meal, so that our brain is continually surprised. An example would be if you had a buffalo mozzarella, some roasted vine tomatoes, a ripe avocado and some warm ciabatta – take a little mouthful of the mozzarella, savour it, then move on to the tomato, savour, then to the avocado, really noticing the textures and the uniqueness of the mouthful; you will find that you come to feel satiated far more quickly and that this feeling stays with you for longer, nicely full, having not eaten too much food. If I could sneak in an analogy that tends to stick in people's mind, eating the same type of food over and over again (for example just having a bowl of pasta and nothing else to play across it) is like always having sex in the same position – it gets boring, the brain switches off! Juggle tastes, textures and savour and so often the weight will come down to where you want it to be.

My final point, which Gemma would love me to mention, is how water can help us feel good, and help us to digest food well, which I believe helps us absorb nutrients from food far more efficiently.

We're less likely to feel uncomfortable digestion-wise, since water can help relieve a sluggish gut as well as help the body glean all the essential vitamins and minerals from those nourishing foods – I like to compare food to one of those Japanese dried tea flowers, which remains closed until it's surrounded by water and then, once you water it, opens up so that the beneficial nutrients within the flower / food can flow and the body can absorb them. I recommend drinking a glass of water every hour – it could be cold or an infusion, such as lemon verbena, fresh mint, or a slice of root ginger in hot water – as this enables the body to adapt and glean all the benefits.

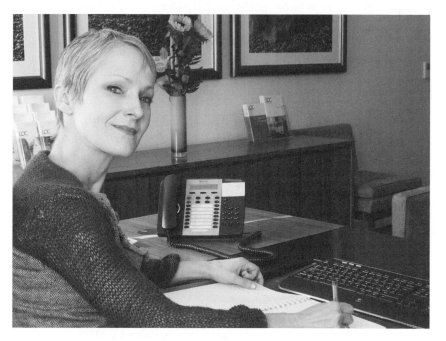

Jane Clarke

Trichology: The Treatment of Hair

GLENN LYONS
Consultant Trichologist

Since my own gorgeous daughter, Caron, lost her seven-year battle with breast cancer in 2004, I have been privileged to meet some incredible survivors of all types of cancer. Sadly, Caron died about four years before so many of the excellent drugs were released on the medical market. Drugs which have given great results and hope to cancer sufferers. One can never give up hope – neither patient nor family - and there is great positivity today about coping and dealing with cancer. GLORIA HUNNIFORD

All my career I have been very aware of the psychological significance of hair. When our hair looks good we feel good. It has an effect on morale, confidence and quality of life. Many people's personalities are identified by their hair; all these are exemplified in the cliché 'a woman's crowning glory'.

Hair grows from small tube-like indentations in the skin called follicles. On the scalp there are 120,000–140,000; blondes tend to have more, redheads less.

Hair growth is cyclic

It has a growing (anagen) phase of 3–5 years at a rate of 1–1.5 cm per month. After this period the hair enters a short resting (catogen) phase of 2–4 weeks before finally entering into telogen, its shedding phase, of 10–12 weeks; this is the 'old' hair we naturally shed on a daily basis.

When we are healthy 90 per cent of our hair is always in the growing (anagen) phase.

Scalp hair can be very sensitive to even mild changes in, for example, metabolism, hormones, nutrition and lifestyle. However, the most profound effect occurs from drug therapy. Their toxic properties very often result in the natural hair cycle being drastically disrupted; the hairs do not enter the telogen (normal shedding) phase as they would normally do but come out very excessively in the anagen phase, sometimes within 4–6 weeks of commencing treatment; it is called anagen effluvium.

Chemotherapy

This describes any treatments where 'chemical' agents are administered, however; all of us relate the word to cancer treatment particularly because of the prevalence and awareness of breast cancer.

From my trichological experience and talking to oncologists and surgeons, the patients' question, 'Am I going to lose my hair?' is of foremost priority, sometimes even before, 'Am I going to live?'

Hair Loss

With certain drugs hair loss will occur in all cases, varying from mild shedding to total hair loss; however, the loss is only *temporary* and full regrowth eventually returns in 99 per cent of patients. Hair loss does not always happen but is dependent on the individual's response to the strength and duration of the treatment.

Some chemotherapy *never* causes hair loss.

There is continual research and advances in chemotherapy and some oncologists are now formulating a 'cocktail' of different drugs whereby it is not always possible to accurately predict as to whether or not hair loss will happen.

Preparing for Hair Loss

The 'cold cap' is adequately described by the author who persevered and found it very beneficial; suffice to say, it does not always reduce hair loss and can cause significant, sometimes unacceptable, discomfort, particularly when initially worn.

Some patients prefer to completely shave their heads *before* their treatment, giving them a sense of control.

I generally advise patients with long hair to have a short style as the hair loss visually will look less; emotionally it may be easier to do this in stages. Other practical ways of coping with hair loss is to wear scarves, hats or ultimately hair pieces or wigs. There are many different styles and colours to choose from and these days they look natural, and are lightweight and comfortable to wear. They are made of either synthetic material or real hair, which is more expensive.

Before considering purchasing, it is essential to go with someone who will give an honest opinion on style and colour suitability.

Wearing these aids *does not* inhibit hair growth but it's advisable to leave them off whenever possible. The scalp tissue will still contain oil and sweat glands so even with total hair loss, daily shampooing is best.

Post Treatment

In some instances the hair texture, colour and shape of the new hair growth are different and on rare occasions can be permanent. It is

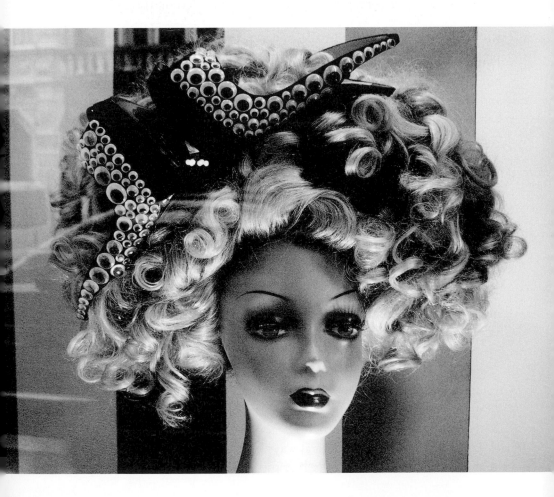

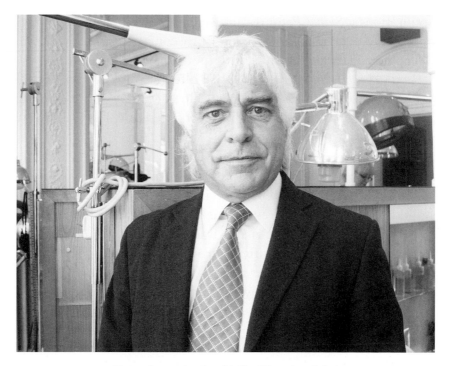

Glenn Lyons in the Philip Kingsley Salon

also often initially fine and fluffy but the follicles eventually produce mature hairs and the rate of growth returns to pre-treatment levels.

Do not massage. The belief that this stimulates hair growth is greatly exaggerated and ultimately could wear away the fine, new hairs.

Other everyday general hair care rules apply.

- Always comb hair when it is wet. Combs are kinder to the hair than brushes and the use of harsh, tightly packed bristle ones should be minimised.
- Avoid using excessive heat from hairdryers and other electrical hairdressing appliances.

As soon as the hair is sufficiently long, usual hairdressing routines such as conditioning and the use of styling products can be resumed. Having your hair styled by a professional hairdresser who knows you and understands your situation can be very helpful and reassuring.

Hair colouring may also be continued, but regardless of previous applications a *Skin / Patch* test must initially be undertaken when chemical colour is going to come into contact with scalp tissue. This is particularly important with 'permanent' hair dyes.

Perms and Highlights do not cause allergies; however, a 'strand test' must also be undertaken on the first occasion after treatment as even though it is new hair it may react differently than previously.

Radiotherapy

All localised radiotherapy can cause hair loss in the treated area. In breast cancer treatment this includes the armpits. When radiotherapy is administered to the head particularly in the treatment of brain tumours it is inevitable that the hair follicles in direct contact are permanently destroyed. However, in many cases hair transplantation can be successfully performed. Like other forms of cosmetic surgery however, it is essential to be referred to the best specialists.

Dentistry: Cancer and the Mouth

PROFESSOR CRISPIAN SCULLY CBE

'Don't fuss, Jeffrey, it's only cancer.'

There were moments when I didn't feel very brave, I was apprehensive about how I would come out of the other end of this tunnel, but my chances of dying on this operating table were very slim. I am actually fitter now than I was before I started my cancer journey.

LADY ARCHER

We all want a healthy mouth which is clean, attractive and painless. This is relatively easy to achieve and maintain, but if you allow hygiene to falter, dental bacterial plaque – a complex biofilm – forms on teeth, and can lead to decay (dental caries with possible pain) and gum disease (gingivitis and periodontitis – with possible tooth loss) as well as halitosis, taste disturbance and jaw-bone problems.

Any mouth problems that may follow chemotherapy may also be aggravated, but there are ways of minimising the effects of chemotherapy by preventing or controlling common oral problems. Maintaining a healthy mouth will help to avoid tooth pain, tooth loss, gingivitis and halitosis and will also help any chemotherapy-related ulcers to heal quickly.

Questions by Gill Heighway

How can decay and gum disease be prevented or controlled?

- brush your teeth at least twice a day using a small-headed medium-hardness toothbrush or an electric toothbrush;
- clean between the teeth by flossing regularly;
- use a mouthwash regularly. Fluoride mouthwashes protect against caries (tooth decay); chlorhexidine and triclosan mouthwashes help to control plaque;
- *Halitosis* (oral malodour) is common in health, on waking in

the morning (*morning breath*) – usually because of low salivary flow and oral cleansing during sleep, although it can also be caused by poor oral hygiene, gingivitis, periodontitis, mouth infections and ulcers. Chemotherapy can also cause mucositis which aggravates halitosis.

How can halitosis be prevented or controlled?

- by brushing your teeth on waking;
- by rinsing the mouth with fresh water;
- by eating;
- by avoiding alcohol;
- by not smoking;
- by eating regular meals;
- by finishing meals with fibrous vegetables and fruits such as carrots and pineapple;
- by avoiding strong-smelling foods such as durian, garlic, onion, spices;
- by eating foods such as cabbage, cauliflower and radish very sparingly;
- by chewing gum, parsley, mint, cloves and fennel seeds;
- by using a mouthwash or proprietary 'breath fresheners';
- by cleaning the tongue with a brush or scraper before going to bed (rather than on waking, which can cause retching;
- by maintaining good oral hygiene generally.

You can suffer from a sore mouth for a number of reasons such as a dry mouth or candidosis (thrush). In particular, mucositis as a result of chemotherapy can lead to ulceration.

How can the risk of sore mouth or ulceration caused by chemotherapy be minimised?

- by sucking ice cubes during some chemotherapy treatments;
- by things such as 'growth factors';
- crucially, by maintaining good oral hygiene;
- by using mouth rinses of benzydamine or the local anaesthetic lidocaine;
- by avoiding eating or drinking for 30 minutes after using the above in order to prolong contact of the drug with the ulcers.

Taste Disturbances   There are five basic tastes: salt, sour, sweet, bitter and umami, but what we call taste in fact is often flavour – a combination of taste with smell (aroma). The sense of taste is mediated by specialised taste buds – mainly on the tongue. These are renewed every ten days, and this can be affected by diet, hormones, age, and factors such as cancer treatments and other drugs. Taste abnormalities can result. However, when people say they cannot taste, it is often that they cannot appreciate the flavour of food and they have often suffered a loss of smell ability rather than taste.

How can taste disturbances be corrected?

- sometimes supplements of zinc or vitamin D can help;
- by chewing food well to increase the release of tastants and saliva production;
- by drinking well;
- by switching different foods during the meal. This can decrease the phenomenon of adaptation and improve taste appreciation.

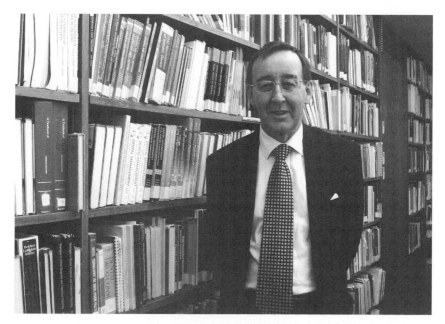

Professor Crispian Scully

Jaw-bone problems (Osteochemonecrosis) Bisphosphonates are drugs injected for the treatment of bone problems in some patients with cancer. Unfortunately they can seriously damage the jaw bone (this is called bisphosphonate-related osteonecrosis of the jaw, or BRONJ) – very similar to the 'phossy jaw' reported in previous centuries as a result of occupational exposure to red phosphorus in makers of matches. Bisphosphonates stay in the bone and have this effect for years or even decades. Prevention is fundamental, since no cure is known.

How can jaw-bone problems (Osteochemonecrosis) be prevented?

- by maintaining good oral hygiene as discussed;
- by avoiding tooth extractions or implant placement, or carrying these out well before being given the bisphosphonates.

Mouth issues specific to breast cancer: There can be mouth side-effects of chemotherapy (CTX) and drugs such as bisphosphonates.

Chemotherapy: Chemotherapy may often cause mucositis and sometimes infections – especially thrush, herpes and human papillomaviruses (HPV). These can be painful, so need treating as discussed. Mucositis is seen especially with CTX using breast cancer drugs such as docetaxel, epirubicin, fluorouracil, idarubicin, mitomycin, mitoxantrone, paclitaxel or vinolrebine.

How can the discomfort caused by mucositis and other mouth infections be reduced?

- by maintaining strict oral hygiene;
- with interventions such as aloe vera, amifostine, granulocyte-colony stimulating factor, glutamine, honey, antibiotic pastille / paste and sucralfate;
- by using a traditional Chinese medicine – Rhodiola algida.

In summary, maintaining strict oral hygiene is critically important in reducing the effects which breast cancer and its treatment can have on the mouth, although there are other measures which can be taken to reduce and minimise specific risks.

A Podiatrist's Perspective

NIGEL TEWKESBURY DPOD MMChS
Podiatrist

When my friend was diagnosed with breast cancer, which she has successfully come through, she said her best advice when reaching the cross roads, is to 'do what the Doctors say'.

DAME KIRI TE KANAWA ONZ DBE AC

I was delighted when Gemma asked me to make a small contribution to her book. I have worked in private practice in London for forty years and it will come as no surprise to learn that I have looked after a number of patients who have undergone chemotherapy for many different types of cancer during this period. Although oncologists do give out a substantial amount of information to patients as to what to expect during treatment, remarkably, many of my patients had no idea that chemotherapy could have an alarming effect on their feet as well as their hands. Skin can become extremely dry and feel very hot and tender with a tendency to crack and peel with redness that gives the appearance of sunburn. Nails on the hands and feet may become very discoloured and brittle and sometimes detach from the nail bed. Ridges and lines across the nails may also appear and there is a potential for bacterial and fungal infections. This is commonly referred to as hand-foot syndrome. In addition, some may experience numbness, tingling and pins and needles in the fingers and toes, although this generally occurs in those with a pre-existing condition such as diabetes, alcoholism and previous chemotherapy treatments.

All said, this may sound pretty grim, but don't despair! There are several things that can be done to help matters and the very best news of all is that practically all of these side effects will resolve in

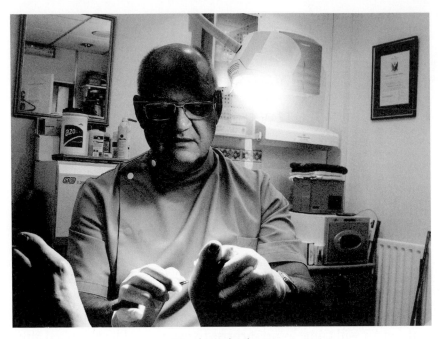

Nigel Tewkesbury

a relatively short period of time when treatment has finished. Addressing dry skin will be one of the most important factors. There is a range of emollient creams available and these should be used extensively. Those containing urea seem to be very effective although everyone will find their own favourite to suit. In the United States, cancer care nurses appear to be unanimous in their praise for Udderley Smooth (R) cream which is becoming more widely available in the UK.

Avoiding hot water is essential as this will exacerbate the red and tender skin. It is a good idea to wear cotton gloves and socks particularly with all that cream being used. Footwear selection becomes a priority as comfort is paramount. Sadly, you will have to temporarily forget those high-heeled Jimmy Choo's and Christian Loubatin's and move to accommodating and soft cushioned shoes. Try keeping insoles in the fridge and popping them into your shoes to cool down your feet. There is no doubt that cold can reduce many of the more painful symptoms affecting both feet and hands.

Looking after your feet is a good thing at the best of times but is especially important during and after chemotherapy. Your podiatrist will be able to help to alleviate many of these irritating symptoms and in particular those relating to problems with skin and nails.

Although I have outlined some of the possible side effects of chemotherapy on hands and feet that I have encountered, not everyone will have these problems. Much is dependent on the treatment regime that is employed and every case is different. Some people undergoing treatment will experience very mild or no symptoms with their feet at all.

It is a privilege to know Gemma as both a patient and a friend. I have been amazed at her resilience and good humour throughout her encounter with cancer and all who read this book will benefit from her experience.

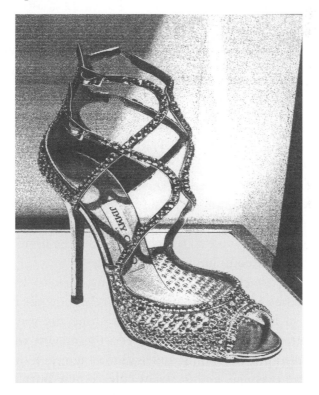

Jimmy Choo shoe 'Falcon' from his Autumn/Winter 2011 Collection

Therapeutic Massage

KELLY READ ITEC

Gemma's book is inspirational. Everyone's story is different and each one in its own way a testament to the human spirit.

KIRSTY WARK

Massage and *Go with the Flow*

When I was asked to write a piece for the book *Go with the Flow* I was really pleased as I feel that at times the role of complimentary therapies in the treatment programme for cancer patients both pre, post and beyond their journey back to full health or for palliative care is undervalued. The complementary therapies can work on the subtle body (the soul, mind and body) and help to nurture and nourish the soul of the patient. They can work on a gentler level, which when the body is stretched to its limit can only do well. When the body is subjected to chemotherapy it not only has the disease to deal with but also the side effects of the chemotherapy itself. Complementary therapies are based upon the premise that the body works as a whole so the holistic body (the mind, body and soul) must be treated to improve well-being.

Therapeutic touch can trace its origins back to the ancient civilisations; the ancient Romans for example knew the benefits of the rituals of bathing and massage, but along the way we seem have forgotten the benefits of touch as a therapeutic medium. In India, for example, the family unit will massage each other in the form of head massage, and in Asian culture new-born babies are massaged on a regular basis for the first year of their life, but in the West we have lost touch with these roots. All too often in this day and age we are cocooned into our own worlds with no contact with other people; with the advent of mobile phones, email etc we communicate with others via these means and many people who live alone do not interact with others on a daily basis. We need contact with others, and we are ingrained with the need for touch in times of ill health or in times of stress . . . How many times have you caught yourself rubbing your temples or neck when in a stressful situation? Or reaching out to someone who has injured themselves? Therapeutic massage is the act of massaging the soft tissues of the body with or without oils (which can be a medium to lessen friction or containing oils which may enhance the benefits of the massage itself).

Disease of the cells of the body, which in turn causes diseases of the body, causes ill health – and massage, as with other alternative therapies, can calm down the body to create a more balanced environment so that self-healing can take place. All too often now-adays, we do not allow ourselves the time or space that our bodies need to cope with modern-day living.

The mind, body and soul are all connected, and chemotherapy has a huge effect on the body as a whole. Yes, side effects may seem to affect only one area of the body, but they do have a knock-on effect.

One of the main areas of concern that I have noticed, when dealing with clients who are having or have completed a course of chemo-therapy; is the overwhelming feeling of tiredness. Massage can help with this symptom greatly, by aiding the client to relax on both a mechanical level (by manipulation, having the muscles relaxed), and a physiological level (allowing the mind to rest for a while).

Feelings of depression and general malaise are also common and with the use of certain essential oils used in the massage medium they can help to lift the mood. Essential oils are oils made from natural items such as plants, barks etc. that are distilled to become highly concentrated and therefore potent, and are not to be confused with fragrances or aromatic oils which have no therapeutic value. In my experience effective oils include camomile, geranium and lavender. Camomile essential oil is fairly floral in its scent and has therapeutic value as a mood lifter. Geranium essential oil again has floral notes, but is less harsh in its scent than camomile; its therapeutic value lies in the fact that it can stabilise the hormones and has a calming effect on the body. Lavender, probably the most recognised scent of the essential oils mentioned, has a slight medicinal scent along with floral undertones; it has a wide range of therapeutic values including being a great anti-depressant. If these

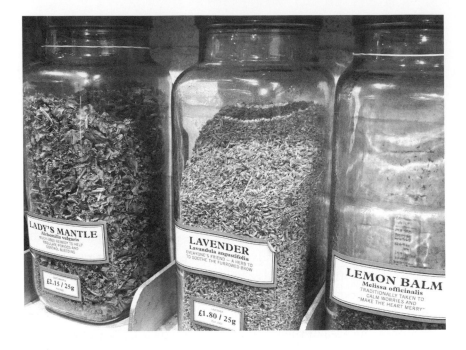

oils are too floral, then also rosemary and clary sage can be used. Rosemary essential oil has a woody scent and is a good mood enhancer, and is also good for combating nausea. Clary sage essential oil has a strong tea-like smell and its therapeutic value lies in the fact that it can lift the mood. These can be blended into a carrier oil (a fatty-based massage oil, such as grapeseed oil) and applied to the body. Only a few drops are needed to have an effect. Also for home care these oils can all be used in the bath, (maximum ten drops placed under the running tap) or in oil burners (maximum five drops placed into the well of the burner and mixed with water to fill the well).

No two treatments will ever be the same – therapeutic massage should not be a cookie cutter treatment whereby the therapist goes through a routine, but it is a tailored treatment for each client at a particular stage in their recovery. The sign of a good therapist is that he or she will 'feel' with his/her hands how the client is on that day – pressure of touch, length of strokes and rhythm will all differ for each treatment. The therapist may pick up on minute changes within the body – change of skin tone, tensing of muscles, flushing of skin, muscular definition etc and work with these subtle ways in which the body is communicating with the therapist.

With massage all the senses should be engaged: touch obviously through the massage itself; sight from a beautifully calming environment; sound from either relaxing music, or total silence; and smell from the oils used. As everyone is individual it is important to ask the client beforehand what their preferences are. But of course one can carry out impromptu treatments anyway.

I met Gemma though my work when she came to me as a client after she had finished her chemotherapy – she was suffering from cramping of the calves and also a tingling of the second and third toes of both feet which felt like pins and needles with a numbness and associated pain in that area. We have devised a course of therapeutic massage based on the legs and feet using general massage oil and I have seen Gemma on several occasions over the course of the last few months. Happily Gemma has given me feedback that the numbness is lessening and I feel this is due to the increase in circulation in the area due to the effects of the massage. I have noted as well that the colour of the skin in the area massage has improved - before the skin had a certain pallor to it, but now the area looks more 'normal'. Also the muscles seem more relaxed in that area. More recently I noted that she had slight swelling in her feet and ankles; Gemma commented that she had not seen her remedial massage therapist that week as usual. This was interesting to see that as she had not had her usual treatment the lymph had collected around the lower extremities causing the swelling. When lymph nodes have been removed the fluid often collects in areas and remedial massage is needed to encourage the lymph to move to the functioning nodes to dispel.

It has been recognised, particularly in the US, that tingling of the legs and feet (peripheral neurology) can be a side effect of some chemotherapy drugs; these symptoms may be short lived or may become a permanent condition after the chemotherapy course has been completed.

It is widely recognised that therapeutic massage can be beneficial in conjunction with allopathic medicine in the care of cancer patients; it can relieve pain, reduce swelling (although it must be mentioned here that areas of lymphedema must never be massaged directly), relieve stress and anxiety caused by the impact of the disease or the treatment plan, help to relieve fatigue and also give the client a much needed break from the treatment plan – a little time just to 'be'. Studies have also suggested that the power of human touch in the form of massage can greatly shorten the time needed to recoup after major surgery. And one must not forget that touch can help the client to re-connect with themselves after surgery / treatment.

I strongly advise anyone wishing to try therapeutic massage within their cancer care plan to find a fully qualified and insured therapist with experience of dealing with clients who have had cancer. Equally important, they must to get advice from their oncologist as whether or not within their journey it would be the right time to try therapeutic massage.

I truly believe that therapeutic massage has a place with easing the effects not of the disease, but of the side effects of the drugs given to fight the disease and for an emotional prop. It also serves as a catalyst for the client whether with palliative care or back to a full state of health when they have travelled along their path.

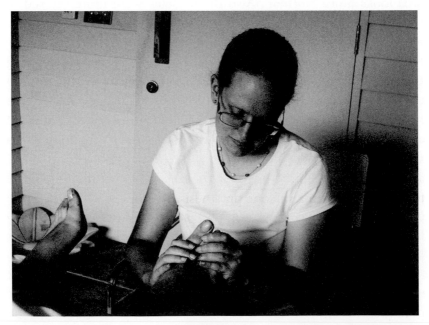

Kelly Read

Fashion and Mastectomy

JUNE KENTON

Fashion underwear and swimwear – Rigby & Peller

It's time we stopped being afraid of cancer – it's like having a wild animal at your throat but with the right attitude and help we can tame it and turn a tiger into a pussycat.

TERRY O'NEILL

Mastectomy! A word that strikes fear into every woman's heart and one that we never want to hear, but we know every day there are women whose lives grind to a halt on learning they have breast cancer and the immediate answer is a mastectomy!

Amongst the multitude of emotions, the shock and the many tears, is also the terror of losing the femininity so vitally important to us as women!

And so it is at this point I will begin the new beginning . . .

Only Two Hours Older . . .

Always remember this. A mastectomy operation takes approximately two hours to complete, which means when you come out of that anaesthetic you are not an old lady – you are only two hours older!

Sadly, in spite of all the caring and gentle approach, you feel like an old lady. Suddenly you find yourself thrown into the world of appliance departments being asked what size bra you wear in order to supply you with a silicone prosthesis.

As 85 per cent of women wear the wrong size bra, it's very likely the prosthesis provided is not going to fit as it should. It moves about, it's difficult to adjust and you are tense and anxious that if you move forward it can be seen, and so, struggling both emotionally and physically and desperately trying to look and feel like you, it's back to the appliance department! And, as you being you again is the all-important criterion, things have to be done in the proper order.

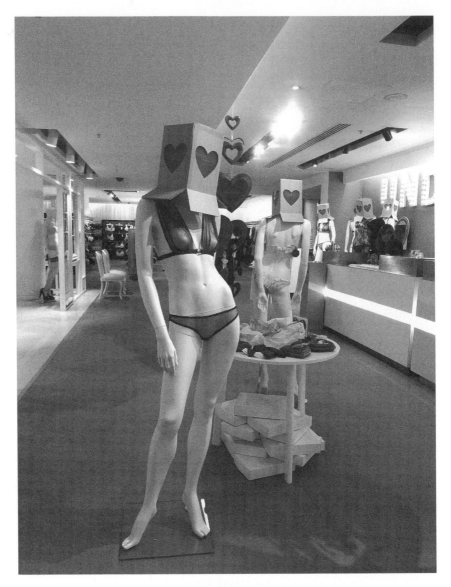

In Selfridges

Rigby & Peller's awareness of breast cancer started as far back as when our shop was called 'Contour' and women who had had mastectomies wore bean bags filled with birdseed inside their bras!

It was also long before I walked the road of breast cancer myself that we had a million breast awareness tickets printed and attached to every bra we sold! I firmly believe each one of us is responsible

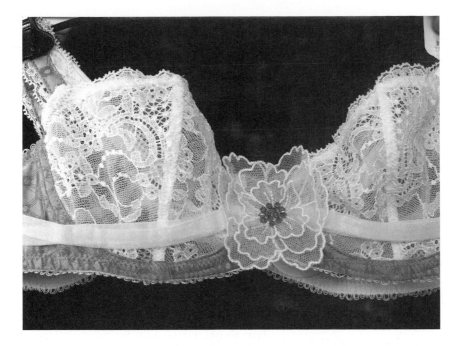

for our own bodies and must have the awareness needed to detect change and act immediately.

At Rigby & Peller we don't believe a prosthesis should be worn in a pocket built inside a bra because very often the bra falls away from the chest wall.

If it fits correctly and the prosthesis is worn close to the chest wall, with the warmth of the skin the bra together with the prosthesis will act as one.

I cannot emphasis enough how imperative it is that a bra fits properly!

Our aim is when a woman who's had a mastectomy wears her bra, she must not only look, but also feel, so confident, it's almost as if it had never happened.

Our shops stock beautiful bras in a multitude of gorgeous fabrics trimmed with lace and ribbons. If the cup size is correct there will be a selection of bras that will hold your prosthesis firmly in place!

We do however recommend no under-wiring whilst healing and again, we carry very pretty bras without wires.

All of our staff are trained to understand not only the physical needs of a mastectomy patient, but also the emotional needs – and I

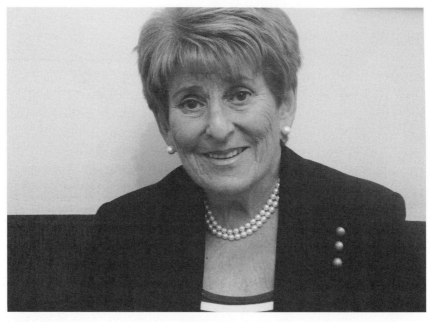

Jane Kenton

will not use that term again because you are not a patient, you are a person! We find very often when a woman comes to us to be fitted with a bra for the first time following the loss of a breast, the one who witnesses her first real tears in public, the one to whom she lets the mask fall, is the fitter in the seclusion of the fitting room!

She's been very brave in front of her family; they are upset enough! 'I'm fine, absolutely fine,' she tells them. To the oncologist 'Thank you yes, I'm coping well,' but it's when she gets undressed in the fitting room she lets go and it doesn't matter how long it takes, how many bras she tries, how often she needs to talk or cry, the fitter is there for her.

Always remember, with the right bra you will confidently walk into any clothes shop just like before and see yourself in a fashion context, not a medical context!

It is at some point following your operation your loved ones may suggest a holiday relaxing in the sun would be a good idea. Immediately you might say 'No, I'm not ready yet. 'I'm still too tired and not up to travelling,' when what you really mean is 'I can't even begin to think about a holiday knowing I can never feel good in a swimsuit again.'

How sad is that, and how untrue!

There are so many swimsuits that will look absolutely wonderful on you, including bikinis! As I previously said we don't have pockets in bras, but we do have them in some swimwear, and I would suggest **not** a prosthesis, but a soft and pliable swim pad be popped into that pocket.

Swimwear with shaped cups would not necessitate a pocket because the swim pad will just sit snugly inside the cup! Top that with a fab matching cover-up – and you are off to the beach or pool looking as gorgeous as you did before!

We are women and we have the right to always feel feminine and special, and our breasts are a major part of our femininity. Just as we wear make-up to enhance our faces, just as we have our hair styled and our nails painted, so we wear the right foundations to add to the attractiveness of our bodies.

A mastectomy does not reduce the value or importance of our body, nor should it reduce how we feel about it!

Be positive about the future, feel confident in that beautiful bra, bikini or swimsuit, and remember a mastectomy takes two hours and you are only two hours older after it – not an old lady!

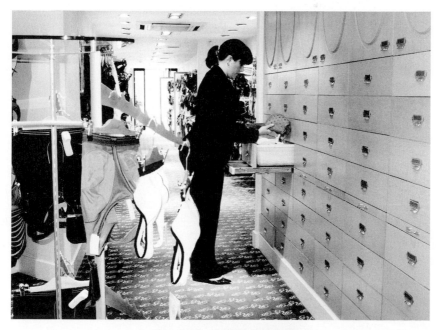

In the shop at Rigby & Peller

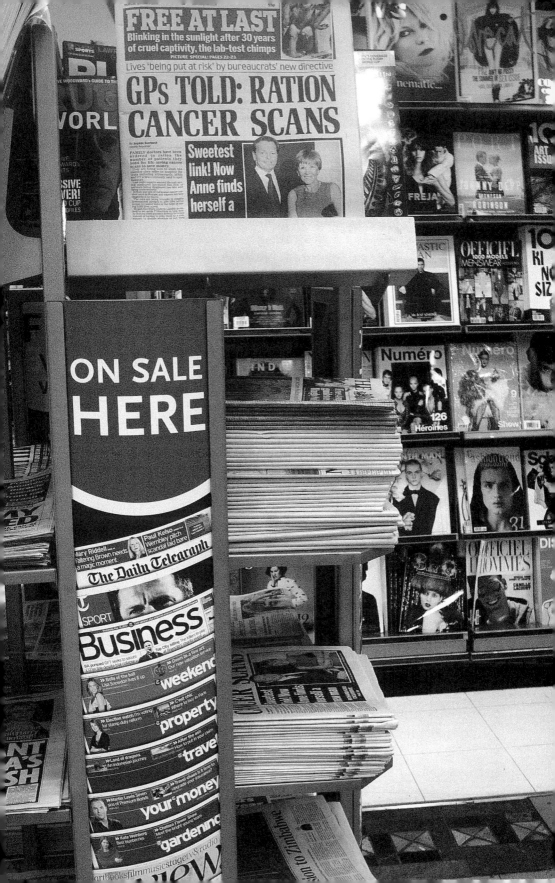

Does the Media Make You Feel Bad about Your Cancer?

DR MIRIAM STOPPARD OBE MD DSc DCL FRCP

The important thing is that people understand that it's a process that has to be gone through, not a ghastly battle that you win or lose.

JOANNA LUMLEY OBE FRGS

A recent study found that more than two thirds of health claims in British newspapers are based on poor evidence. So much of the media aims to create horror stories, irrespective of science and evidence, that it's often difficult to hang on to a balanced view.

For every statistic that paints a black picture, however, there's one that reads more optimistically. Alongside a depressing outcome one can invariably cite a hopeful one. I'm in the business of hope and optimism and take seriously my job of analysing and critiquing the statements of scaremongers and the claims of doom merchants.

I'm often faced by a dilemma. Many people feel more comfortable with and are more ready to accept stories, be they positive or negative, than scientific facts – single case studies, personal histories, what scientists would call anecdotal evidence and, though interesting, rightly dismiss as not worth the paper it's written on.

But stories are dramatic and emotional and slip into the public consciousness never to be erased. Not by science, not by evidence and certainly not by statistics. The person who likes personal stories is flummoxed by incidence rates: 1 in 80 – the rate for twin pregnancy; 1 in 200 – the number of people who have psoriasis; 25 per cent – the increase in birth rate from 600,000 to 750,000 per annum. Percentages are anathema to the person who wants stories. This makes the job of presenting hard evidence in an accessible way a taxing one.

Here's the world I work in – a brainteaser posed by some US

researchers examining how well lay people understand statistics. Participants were told that the chance of muscle breakdown after taking a statin is 4 in 10,000 and the chance of liver inflammation is 1 in 100. Only 40% correctly understood that muscle breakdown is less common. The rest only saw that four is bigger than one so thought muscle breakdown was the greater risk.

Presenting an accurate, sensible picture is nowhere more difficult than in cancer. Besides the scare stories that must be tempered there are rafts of advice which are simply daft. I can see for a cancer patient – a non-scientist who is besieged by doubts and fears – it's well nigh impossible to skein out what to take seriously and what to ignore. What's distorted and what isn't? What's hyperbole and what's objective? Who can I trust?

It's tempting for anyone in the throes of cancer treatment to think, well, it might help so I'll risk it. But then, how do you assess risk? We're into more deep water here. You may read headlines that taking HRT will double your risk of breast cancer. Let's look at the figures.

In 2003 a study of over a million women estimated that there'd be 19 extra cases of breast cancer if 1000 women took combined (oestrogen and progestogen) HRT for 10 years. In 2005 this figure was revised down to an extra 12 cases. In 2008 the figure went up to three extra cases per year. In 2010 a UK study conducted by Bristol University failed to show any increased risk at all. One thing's for sure – your risk of getting breast cancer if you take HRT isn't double. It's a small additional risk and much smaller than, say, the increased risk of failing to have your first baby before you're 30. That is double.

Good data, I mean robust data that stands up to scrutiny, is hard to find in the media. Good interpretations, even harder. Where would you search? Sadly the internet is a dangerous place. There's no hierarchy of information. Bad information rubs shoulders with good. Crazy pseudo-science jostles with high-class, evidence-based research. It's hard to sort out the wheat from the chaff.

There are ways to thread a path through the morass of websites, blogs and self-help gurus. In general terms medical association websites are reliable. Cancer Research UK is one. Those run by doctors and scientists like NetDoctor are objective. Prestigious clinics like the Mayo Clinic can be relied upon. Patient associations serving the needs of people with a particular complaint likewise.

If it's balanced opinion you're after there aren't many places to look. It takes a brave communicator to come out against prevailing medical opinion. For instance, there have always been questions about the effectiveness of mammography screening for breast cancer but I've remained an advocate. Recently, the results of a large study showed that screening does not improve the death rate from breast cancer. Critics claim screening leads to overdiagnosis and wastes money. This doesn't stop me supporting breast screening. No one died of overdiagnosis – but underdiagnosis kills.

The antidote to bad science is good science. Eschew rogue sources. Reject any without proper qualifications and membership of recognised professional bodies. Cultivate scepticism about florid media reporting and outlandish claims. Establish a direct line to a doctor you trust who will act as a corrective to media scare tactics, myth and folklore.

Knowing what to believe isn't made easier when doctors appear to renege on previous advice: red wine first protects against heart disease then it doesn't (it does); eggs raise your cholesterol then they don't (they don't); overuse of mobile phones promotes brain tumours then it doesn't (it doesn't). These turnarounds aren't capricious. It's unintelligent to ignore new science. Such information demands a change of tack so don't lose heart.

Several givens are emerging in the field of cancer that most patients can rely and act on. Vitamin D3 appears to be canceroprotective so supplements are worth taking. I don't think it's an overstatement to say that obesity is cancerogenic so staying a healthy weight is important. Exercise stabilises practically every system in the body so a daily brisk walk for half an hour should be the rule, and general pottering about rather than sitting around.

Without being pernickety, diet is worth thinking about. Any food eaten fresh is preferable to eating it cooked. Don't stop at five a day – eat 12–14. Antioxidants, the cancer killers, are found in the highest concentration in dark coloured foods. The darker the colour the more antioxidants. So eat the darkest green leaves you can find and the blackest fruit – blueberries are good. Eat nuts and seeds, full of vitamins, antioxidants like selenium and essential fatty acids. On that subject you could chase down foods rich in omega-3s, foods like fatty fish (salmon, herring, sardines) and even take a daily supplement. And make a friend of fibre.

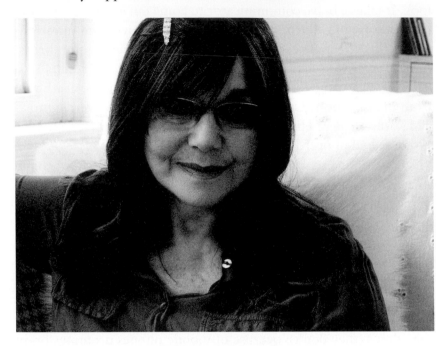

Miriam Stoppard

Where Are Faith and Community in all of this?

RABBI DAME JULIA NEUBERGER DBE

In experiencing the march of science, Gemma's keenness to share her experience with us all is spirited, helpful and most welcome. With the new phase in her life, a tragic brush of sadness will drain us, while revealing at the same time, the alternative gifts of life.

THE RT HON THE BARONESS BETTY BOOTHROYD OM PC

And God said, 'Let us make man in our image, after our likeness . . . ' So God created man in his own image; in the image of God created He him; male and female created He them.'   (Genesis 1:26–7)

We human beings have a strong consciousness of our bodies, not least because of the idea that we have been created in the image of God. What then happens, if we feel that we are in God's image, when cancer eats away at us and we have surgery to remove the offending part of the body? What does that say to us about our body image in God's image, and what does it say to us about a part of us rebelling, and turning against us?

For many people with cancer, coming to terms with what has happened spiritually and emotionally is enormously hard. That is at least in part because much of the initial period of diagnosis, tests, more diagnosis;, and then decisions about surgery, radiotherapy and chemotherapy, are made very quickly. The emotional support, if it is provided within a healthcare slotting, is slower to materialise in most cases, and the spiritual support is often non-existent in that setting, with rabbis, priest, imams, and others often at a loss for words about what to say. That is partly because spiritual care, though accepted as a necessary part of healthcare more or less universally in the western world, has very little attention paid to it, few resources, very little in the way of human resources, and almost no training, other than the very specialised training for healthcare chaplaincy, largely pioneered by the Reverend Walter Smith and others in the United States.

So what are the things we should be thinking about? First, a change in self-image. I started deliberately with body image. For women with breast cancer, losing either a part or the whole of a breast, the change in body image is combined with a change in sexual allure, or perception of sexual allure. Often, women feel 'incomplete', and they are worried about partners and husbands seeing them as 'incomplete', somehow 'desexed', women. Add into that an idea that we are, in some way, in the divine image and for many women, and also for men who have disfiguring surgery to cut out a cancer, the sense of wholeness, of completeness, of being a little bit in the image of the divine, starts disappearing.

Many people think that our doubts and uncertainties about our faith in the face of frightening disease are because of the question about why such a thing should have happened to us, on the basis that we are 'good people'. That idea rests on the idea of reward from God for behaving well, and punishment for behaving badly – and it is true that some sections of all religious faiths strengthen that view. But all religious faiths also have within them important ideas about just and good people suffering for no particular reason, or maybe as a test. Take Job, for instance in the Hebrew Bible. He was truly afflicted, had all sorts of diseases, lost all he had, and was mocked by his friends. But the lesson is not that he was a bad person, being punished. Rather, it is that he was a good person, and through it all he did not lose his faith. So the first, and important, test is keeping faith when terrible things are happening to you. And one can only do that by not regarding the cancer as a direct punishment from God, but instead something that happens in our bodies, where cells get out of control, where human beings have searched – with God's gift of intelligence – for cures and alleviation, and may not have come up with the magic bullet yet. But this is about human failure – and also about human skills, and human devotion, rather than about God's punishment.

So one strong message that spiritual care givers need to give is that the cancer (or any other disease) is not a reason for giving up on God. Indeed, it might be a reason to hang on ever more strongly,

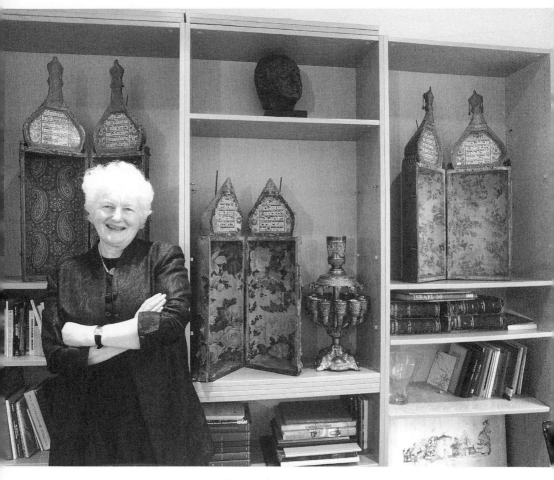

Julia Neuberger

even a bit grimly, when life is tough– because belief in God also allows us to believe in the skills and devotion of those who are trying to help, and helps us see things in a more rounded way. It helps us to see we are very small parts of a much bigger picture, and that it is unlikely that God would just send us – individually – a disease to punish us. For some of us, it might seem like something to test us, and justify us taking it on as a real 'fight'– looking the cancer in the eye and saying we won't be vanquished, or seeing it as a test of our resolve to do anything, anything we possibly can, to get better, to rout the cancer, to defeat this alien invader. Both the fight, and the sense of gratitude and recognition of God in those who are trying to help, make us able to see God as the source of wisdom, of skills, of the human intelligence, of the desire by human beings to do more research, to learn more, to treat more, as well as the source of human strength and determination, and sheer bloody-mindedness! And that sense of God's presence in the intelligence and devotion of our doctors, nurses and carers also allows us greater humility in our dealings with those who are trying to help.

But the second element goes back to our bodies and our image of ourselves. 'Who am I when I have lost half a leg, a breast, am having chemo, and have lost my hair? The answer, as I am fighting my cancer, is that I am just the same person, afflicted certainly, but fighting to survive, trusting my carers, and learning more about myself in the process. I am learning what I can cope with – and never thought I would. I am learning about the nature of courage and resignation. I am learning about pain – and pain is not some-thing that ennobles the spirit, and is to be avoided – and I am learning about the immense skills and devotion of those specialists who deal with pain, who remove it from me without leaving me like a zombie. I am learning that the absence of a breast may have shocked me – and others – in the short term, but is as nothing compared with what others have to have removed. I am learning that I can continue to love, think, work, create, and indeed make and maintain close friendships when I have lost part of me. I am learning that there is another side to me, a side less in thrall to the physical me, but more in touch with my inner self. I am learning – if I am religious – to trust God although I hate what is happening to me. If I am not religious, but have a spiritual sense, I am feeling my spirit being tested by all this, but I am coming to a form of resolution that is making me clearer about what matters to me, and what is froth and unimportant. Indeed, though I would far rather not have gone through any of this, I am beginning to think I am a better person, more in touch with what really matters, than before it all started.'

All those sentiments in that last paragraph are a composite of what people have said to me over many years dealing with cancer, or other life-threatening illnesses. Most – not all – have gone through a stage of anger and fear and have come to a mixture of fighting for survival, fighting against the disease, and a better sense of themselves. Most, but not all, have found some sense of meaning and closeness to God in what has happened to them. And most never thought that would be the case at the beginning. So what we need is to develop far better skills in the giving of spiritual support and care to people with cancer and other frightening illnesses. It should not all be provided by rabbis, priests, imams, pundits and Buddhist sisters and monks, because not all people have a specific faith. They too will need – and should receive – spiritual care. We need to grow our skills here, and learn from the people who have gone through the serious illnesses, the changes in body image, the sense of relinquishing what does not matter, and we should use what they can teach us to provide better support and care for the next generation.

I have learned more over my lifetime from trying to support people with serious illness, some of whom are facing their end, than from any other group of people. What we learn is humbling. But what we also learn is that spiritual care is important, and that people's spirituality, when facing serious illness, takes a knock, but also becomes something many people, if not most, want passion-ately to explore and learn from. And the message from all that is that the human spirit, founded on belief or even not, especially when supported and cared for by others, is immensely strong.

Where Is God in all of this?

THE REV. CANON DR JAMES WOODWARD

ST GEORGE'S, WINDSOR

The very word 'cancer' automatically triggers dread and fear. Everyone prays that it will not be them or their partner, children or friends that get invaded. The truth is, the odds are getting better and the medical profession and cancer research can and will destroy this enemy.

The centres for care and research will need every support possible, both personal and financial. Those of us who are fortunate to be in good health now should be so very grateful – just for today.

DAVID SUCHET CBE

Illness is a threat to our whole being, our individuality, all that we live for and hope for, all that gives us pleasure and satisfaction. Our body and our will struggle with the experience. We want to fight and shout.

No one can quite foresee what will happen to them in life. Our living has an unpredictability and fragility about it. Nowhere is this better demonstrated than in illness. Disease is a part of our world and for many it becomes a part of their living and their dying. For some it comes with advancing years, and highlights the unforesee-ability of a life that naturally draws to its close. For others illness strikes randomly and unpredictably. It is no respecter of age, of class, of our system of fairness and justice as individuals and as a society. One moment a person enjoys physical health and well-being and the next they face some kind of challenge to their physical and spiritual stability and equilibrium. There is no one way of looking at illness. It is a mystery which in the end eludes all our attempts at comprehension and explanation. Our task here is to discern the mystery and meaning of illness. It is to ask how we might find God in illness, and whether the experience can be viewed as a phase of life, with its own time, significance and meaning.

So, to look for some kind of meaning in our shared apprehension of suffering may be to begin a journey of exploration of faith. To find God in illness may be a stepping-stone to building a better world. To attend to the experiences of illness may lead us on a journey of change and movement that enables us to live each day to the fullest as a gift, by being honest with ourselves and fully human in our loving and in our praying.

On our journey into life we should allow what we are given to shape us, mould and form us; for these experiences are the building blocks of our salvation.

It is important, however, not to be dishonest about the darker side of the reality of illness. There is here deep tragedy, horror and awfulness. Illness makes both patient and bystander feel the depth of loss and pain. Some feel so overwhelmed by illness that the darkness is unquenchable. For others there are few answers to their questions.

Many look at illness in an attempt to find some meaning, and wonder where responsibility lies. Are sin and disease related as cause to effect? Is disease a punishment for those things in our lives that are amiss? This is one natural and understandable response to our search for meaning within illness.

But both common sense and our Christian picture of God teach us to reject any direct relation between our conduct and illness and to reject the idea of illness as divine punishment: it is all too random for that. It is true, however, that our own wholeness in living is intimately inter-connected with others. There are many causes of illness and the illness of an individual often reflects a corporate or social disease, as when asthma is induced by pollution of the air. Some are denied the possibility of health and well-being because of their working conditions or their living conditions and environment.

So to ask the reasons for illness is natural. There are other responses too. In the novel *Silence*, by Shusaku Endo, an old priest who suffered much says to God, 'Lord, I resented your silence.' The answer he received was simple and profound: 'I was not silent, I suffered beside you.' We may never know comprehensively what causes illness, but what we can affirm is God's presence in all situations. This is a journey to acceptance and surrender, not just as an attitude but as a different way of living. In the questions about meaning it is important to stand back as we attempt to embrace the mystery, the paradoxes, the uncertainties and the ambiguities of the causes and meanings of illness. Maybe, try as we will, we shall never be able to discern much meaning in illness and have to endure this lack of meaning. But in the search for patterns and pictures we need to be aware of the danger of bringing inappropriate meaning into the picture and avoid, if we can, over-simplified ideas when we introduce issues like judgement or punishment.

These questions are often asked by bystanders. Very often those who have to learn to befriend illness know that there are no easy answers and become voluntary painbearers, absorbing anger and hurt and giving back to us acceptance and care. In this process they allow what is given to them to shape them, not for ease, but for glory, in a humble, trusting and forgiving attitude.

So all of us are fragile: a mixture of weakness and compassion. Perhaps part of our journey into or around illness is to find a way of making good those parts of our lives that are painful or just meaningless. A writer who spent many years reflecting on God, Julian of Norwich, said, 'Love was our Lord's meaning.' In this context perhaps part of our encounter is to try and serve the purposes of love in our living and through our illness. In this search, we may find God. We may find that there is the possibility of becoming whole by our experiences and our relationships.

One of the core issues that emerges is our search for meaning as we begin to think about what it means to be human. God is interested in every aspect of our lives and it may be necessary to explore where God is in the dimensions of our lives, so that we can discover and rediscover the truth about life, ourselves and God. As God has taken on our human lives, in Christ, it is within our experience that his grace moves and works. So what are the things that we might learn as we find a way through this experience?

The first is that we may learn to wait. As illness imposes its enforced rest upon us, we must never underestimate the essential dignity that belongs to the 'patient'. From being an active person who does lots of things, the patient suddenly becomes someone to whom things are done, not only carried along by unfamiliar routines, but quite possibly unable to do the things which were once easy. There is much to be learnt from the experience of passivity in our attitude both to time and to life. We may, for

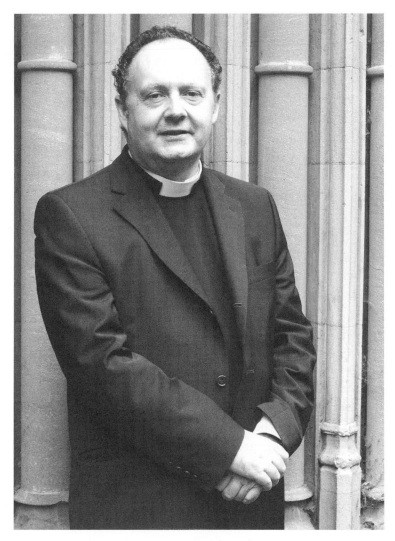

James Woodward

example, value people for who they are, rather than what they do. We may also, inevitably and with all its difficulties, have to learn to suffer. One of the difficulties that many doctors labour under is a range of unrealistic expectations that they can make this better and take all of the pain away. This, surely, is only partly true. Those who are ill teach us that there is no pain-free existence and that it is unlikely that any of us will remain unaffected by the pain of living and dying. This suffering may take a variety of forms but in the end we shall have to face it, live with it, and learn to handle it. Within the dependence of illness we have to learn both to receive and to give. Sometimes it can be very difficult to be vulnerable with people and receive what they have to offer to us. In the acuteness of illness we can be overwhelmed by the small tokens of kindness expressed through a variety of people.

If we are unable to give materially in our illness then we have to learn other ways of giving. This is about the quality of the present moment in the way we look and see and respond to people. It may also involve expressing some things to whose we care about and love, perhaps things that the activity and health of our lives have never given us the opportunity to express. In the business of an active life so much of the force and meaning of our lives and relationships can remain unspoken. Now may be an opportunity to give through expressing those things that have remained lost or hidden, hopes and fears, regrets or feelings of thankfulness.

Within the context of all this learning, for those who are ill, bystanders or professional carers, there is an undergirding learning that we must continue to participate in. We all need to work together in learning to serve. This involves sensitivity, attentiveness, a desire to listen carefully and lovingly to those who are most vulnerable and in need.

It means building a better world by the quality of our listening and connecting in the present. It is about giving our time and resources to look after those who are most vulnerable within our community and society.

So where do we find God and how do we find God? God as the Creator, as a circle of love within which there is movement, holds together the tensions of our experiences. In the space between pain and illness, suffering and death, faith and fear, hope and despair, tears and laughter, God is there as ultimate value, a mystery that can and will inspire and renew us.

This is not to deny that illness poses genuine difficulties for belief. There are, perhaps, irreconcilable contradictions between human experience and what we are able to believe. However, part of the discovery of God in illness is to move to a point of acceptance, for acceptance contains within it an attitude of heart and mind which can enable people to enhance the meaning and purpose of their own lives and the lives of others. It is within this process, in the experience of life in all its complexity, that the gift of God is present and discovered.

One of the surprises of working closely with those who are ill is seeing how they become aware of how blessed their lives are. They face their pain but also have a sense of the wonder and loveliness of life. Small kindnesses bring people to tears as they ponder the preciousness and delight of living. To realise the love of neighbours and friends through flowers and visits and concern makes for fuller, deeper, more complete living. It is within this exploration of death that God is present, bringing people together, building bridges and healing wounds.

This experience of God as present, as with us, can deepen faith in love and compassion and bring to life a sense of awe, intricacy and balance. Sometimes it is necessary to strive to reach this point: illness can throw us off balance in the matter of faith as in the rest of life.

God is seen and experienced in the glory of creation, in both its beauty and its absurdity. God is present in both the thistle and the rose, the slug and the butterfly, the crow and the blackbird. They are all part of the same concert. There is also glory in the anger, pain and loneliness because God puts these in the kingdom as part of a delicate and complex structure and relationship. We are all part of God's creation, created, redeemed and liberated by the love of God and by seeing glory in others. In this sense we reflect the words of Irenaeus, an early Christian writer: 'The glory of God is a human being fully alive.'

This is a God who is faithful and wants us to grow to maturity through our mutual cooperation, trust and obedience. The discovery of this God is through an awareness of God's love at work within us. In this sense nothing can separate us from this presence and God continues to offer to transform all illness, evil and pain through all of our experiences and responses. We find God in our prayer, in our offering, in our patience, in our questions and in our perseverance.

The discovery of God's presence in illness is an awareness of the grace, truth, goodness, love, beauty and peace of our living and striving and hoping. Finding God in illness is part of an affirmation that God is glorified in the whole range of our human inter-connectedness, but above all in those who are sick for they have nothing to give but themselves, aware of weakness and vulnerability.

Breast Cancer – A Journey: Part Two, A Year Later

GEMMA LEVINE

I went with the flow which carried me through. I looked at the angel eyeball to eyeball, one of us blinked and it wasn't me, I refused.

THE CHIEF RABBI, LORD JONATHAN SACKS

October 2010 – September 2011

'Hello, you're back! Are you awake?' My sister Sally hung her head, eyes diverted whilst my friend Zelda peered over my bed anxiously, and both faces stern. Oh, my God am I alive? Ooo-aw, I feel awful, the right side of my body felt as though it was missing. The pain was indescribable. There were so many attachments by my side, drips and anaesthetic equipment, I couldn't move. 'Oh! You're both still here! How long was I in surgery?' ' A couple of hours, I heard them utter. I was very drowsy but managed to stutter one final question before I lapsed into heavy sleep. 'Did I – eh – eh – have the mastectomy?' They hesitated; the answer was 'Yes.' Disquiet, despair but resignation took hold of me, then a void.

*   *   *

Two weeks before I went into hospital, papers arrived in the post and one was from my surgeon, Professor Mokbel to my GP Dr Nazeer. It read, 'I have discussed with her [me] the proposed surgery, which will entail right total mastectomy and axillary node clearance . . . '

This information shocked me; we all have a central fear. Somehow I had to come to terms with the fact that I would have one breast entirely removed in order for the disease to be obliterated. It was the only thing to be done, there were no options. It was not easy. Nights went by when I could not sleep, only dozed, from extreme exhaustion.

Friday 15th October 2010 arrived. It was a grim, drab, grey morning and together with my sister Sally, we went to the Princess Grace Hospital. The automatic doors sprung open as we walked through early, in preparation for my operation later in the day.

I was terrified.

I have a vague recollection of that day as I was in denial of the fact that my body would change and that I would have only one breast. No one should tell you 'there are worse things'. Yes, of course there are, but the individual in question has to live with the knowledge that a private and sensual part of one's body has been removed. Does it affect one's womanhood? I think that as I am seventy-one years old, it has happened at a time in my life that I can overcome, but I hasten to add, age is an arguable factor to everyone. I feel that, for me, had this occurred during my younger years, it would have been inconceivable.

My stay at the hospital lasted three nights. I am afraid I cannot say anything wonderful about the care. So much so, that in the numbness of the night, shortly after my operation and awaking abruptly in panic, I could not alert a nurse. I could not get out of bed, nor reach for a light or a call button. I felt marooned and alone. I called my son in America to telephone 'the powers that be' at the hospital, in order to arouse some attention. It was very distressing. A good hour after the call, a night porter arrived then a nurse. Finally I was attended to.

The three days in the hospital passed, without a major incident and I became engaged in the pedestrian routine. I was helpless and became accustomed to indulging in the recognition, perspective and trajectory of my life.

I recall that the most welcome moment regarding my stay was signing the 'exit' sheet. I felt very weak and needed assistance dressing. I could not face a mirror and look at my body. As from that day onwards to this day, I have not summoned up the courage.

As soon as I said 'goodbye' to the day nurses and had a brief breakfast, I left the hospital as weak as a kitten, and was bundled into my sister's car. What an angel she was, stopping off on the way home at Prêt à Manger for a slice of my favourite carrot cake, to cheer me from the shattering ordeal of major surgery!

Later that morning, I was given a huge treat to celebrate

my homecoming. My friend Jeremy King, owner of the Wolsley Restaurant, sent a taxi at noon, to my apartment. The delivery included two large crates. Packed inside was a three-course lunch of my choice, together with china, glassware, napkins, and garnish for all courses! This was a gift I will never forget. My friend and I sat down for an hour in comfort, before I retired to bed exhausted.

The operation came and went. The surgeon was satisfied that he had removed the cancer; as far as I was concerned that was all that mattered. I spent days after the operation at home and was cosseted by the constant care of family and friends. My fridge was filled; my chores were done; flowers were delivered constantly on the doorstep. Tears welled in my eyes for the overall concern. People came to see me. Some from abroad and other friends I had not seen for years seemed to close the circle of a lifetime. I was fortunate. My sister said, 'Make the most of this time, it won't last.' She was right!

There were several side effects and a few downsides to the last few months. I noticed that my eyebrows and eyelashes disappeared. I asked my friend Madhu, what should I do? 'Oh, go to Boots, they have the perfect remedy, RapidLash.' She was right, within a few weeks of application, they were back as normal. Then, my finger nails split halfway down the base of the nail bed. That problem I am still addressing even months later, but have faith they will grow back to normal strength, given time. I found that my middle toes on my left foot became numb and when walking with shoes, I was forced to stop as it was often painful. This problem, after tugging at my toes and a little self-massage became easier. At a later stage, I did go to Kelly Read for a foot massage, which did wonders!

My hair is good, as I explained in my introduction. The strength and condition were, in my view, totally due to the 'cold cap'. What a bonus! What an invention! I reiterate a huge relief.

My skin became dry, but with regular cream application, it was back to normal in no time. The excellent creams I used and still do are *Aqueous cream BP* for the scar tissues and for general use for dry skin, *Vaseline essential moisture lotion.*

Perhaps one of the most important problems that occurred was that I lost concentration when reading. I found I could read and reread a page or paragraph and still was unaware of the content. I find now, eighteen months later, that I can actually finish a book and have no concerns whatsoever about my concentration. (It could be the choice of book!)

I think one of the worst side effects is that, emotionally, sustaining my equilibrium is at its lowest. I become upset too regularly, Reading a letter or taking part in an unpleasant conversation, my reactions are exaggerated. I become nervous and agitated beyond reason.

Having only one breast provides a problem with clothes, especially underwear. From the hospital I was given brochures and websites. I tried ordering mastectomy bras from mail order and failed and was constantly sending the garments back. I then discovered a local store that personally attended to me and provided me with the correct size bra and correct 'pads' to place inside. I was told that when packing your suitcase, it was advisable to pack your prosthesis in your main luggage as the metal content could set off alarms! Swimming also presented a problem. I was worried that when swimming, the pad would fall out, float away on the surface of the pool, hit someone in the face and this could be so embarrassing! I found a solution to the problem: by not using a pad, by simply not caring what other people thought. I am sure no one noticed as I enjoyed my swim and threw my cares to the wind!

Radiotherapy was for me a frightening and terrifying experience. Even though time spent under radiation was not long, the process of accommodating to the correct position was, at times, lengthy and painful. Emotionally, it was similar to a torture. I was stretched on the bed, naked from the waist upwards, with my right arm aloft, strapped into a brace. As the operation on my right breast was recent, my body was adjusting to the enormity of the incision, and my skin felt as though it was being torn apart. Lying in that position, as the technicians were adapting the control and angle of the machine, I gritted my teeth and prayed that the location of the machine was on the correct spot and this critical invasion would be concluded as soon as possible.

The 'Varian Trilogy Machine' took approximately fifteen minutes to set up; pen marks, like a temporary tattoo, were carefully impressed on my skin, a little like the markings one sees on pavements before the paving stone is dug up. After a further ten minutes, the awesome large silver grey dome of the machine started to steer itself from left to right and dominate the specific area of the body that had been infested with the cancer. I heard a cold voice saying 'Remain absolutely still' followed by the clicking of heels as the radiologists rushed out of the room. I closed my eyes. All I could hear was a continuous chant, 'chaaah-chink' then click, then 'chuc-ugh' then click. This was the governing sound which persisted until the cycle had concluded. My mind mused with visions of ethereal mists surrounding the Swiss Alps. The mists covered everything, changing by the moment. Out of the mists arose shapes, just half images which created the foundations of half dreams. A while later, fifteen or twenty minutes, my fleeting dreams were interrupted by a sing-song voice, 'All over for today.' A moment that could not have been more welcome. 'See you tomorrow, Gemma.'

There is no question that radiotherapy exhausts you. A rest during the day is essential. The spasmodic feeling of sharp burning pains on the area is something one has to get used to. But as the weeks went by, the pains gradually eased. I felt far more discomfort and pain during this period, than during chemotherapy.

No sooner had I begun to feel stronger, I discovered I had swelling in my right fingers, hand and arm, I paid a visit to my surgeon and was told I had lymphoedema, because of an abnormal build-up of fluid called lymph in the body tissues, which occurred when part of the lymphatic drainage system had been removed by surgery. Alternatively, it could possibly be damaged by radio-therapy treatment. I was told this condition could be with me for life. Immediately I was sent to a remedial specialist, Bernie Martin.

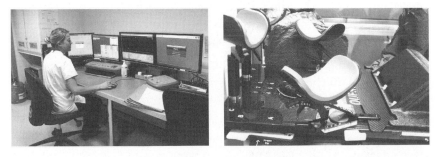

The radiographer's viewing console and the arm support
braces for radiotherapy

The treatment I am receiving on a regular basis, weekly, gives me comfort and if I am lucky, an Irish or Jewish joke to soften the pain! I was told I had to wear an elasticised compression sleeve and give

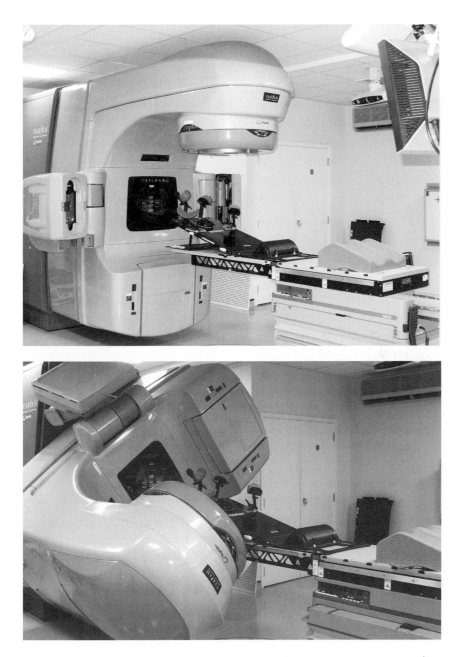

The Varian Trilogy Machine

myself appropriate gentle exercise as often as possible. The sleeve I wear all day and every day controls the fluid in the lymph glands. I remove it at night and for showering and swimming. I swim every day which helps enormously. I firmly believe this is the most rewarding discipline and, again, compiled my own exercises. In the heat of the summer, the weight together with the texture of the sleeve is unbearable, but I have to 'go with the flow'! At night, I take four pillows and form a barricade. I place the affected right arm elevated on to the pillows. After several months now, I have become accustomed to this strange way of sleeping. The trick is to arrange the pillows for your own comfort before settling; otherwise they fall on the floor!

Having this oedema condition is unfortunate and not easy to deal with. Firstly, one's clothes do not fit, because of the swollen arm and the elasticised compression sleeve. I cannot wear any tight-fitting garments. I am forced to select loose-fitting coats, jackets and raglan sleeve sweaters. In this case you can always say to your husband /partner, 'Let's shop 'til I drop!' A terrific excuse? I have become very sensitive to people's comments as to how I look. I think the most irritating one is 'You look good – considering.' Why they have to add, 'considering'. I will never know! Dis-heartening to say the least! It is an upset and constant reminder of cancer which one wants to forget. But feeling sorry for yourself does not help. A waiter in a restaurant in Venice said to me, 'Your arm is a reminder that you are lucky and still here, to live, see and take the best out of life.'

Let's take a break: I think this could be a good moment to tell you one of Bernie Martin's Jewish jokes:

> *A Jewish man, Hymie, desperately ill on his sick bed in hospital, calls for the Rabbi to say a few words of comfort. Rabbi says, 'Hymie, I am so sorry to see you this way. But are you comfortable?' Hymie with a shrug of his shoulders says, 'Well – I've got a couple of shops in Golders Green!'*

My self-esteem was shattered at the occasional party. I found it difficult and tiring to stand in a crowd and chat with a glass in one hand, wine spilling over as my hand shook from nerves. I became overheated, my clothes stuck to me and my hair became moist. I was not at my best. I needed to sit down, but thought I would be conspicuous. Parties, I decided, were not for me at this time. I had the same experience at an art exhibition, a concert and theatre. I became weak with the strain. But the months go by and one regains one's confidence; we go with the flow.

Sitting in the sun, which I love, I was advised to do so in moderation. Apparently the sun is good for the skin for a short period, providing you use a good sun protection cream. I have to sit with my arm resting in an upward position and propped up high so as not to allow any pressure on the upper arm. It is quite comfortable but one has to get used to it.

What is the good news under these circumstances? People do notice the sleeve. It is made in a skin-tone colour but is not too unsightly. I have found that people detect this and ask to carry my bags, open doors for me and in some cases I am offered a seat on a crowded bus! When travelling abroad, I now arrange to have a wheelchair at the airport. At busy airports this is a 'must'. I am taken through queues and crowds, through passport checks and security. I arrive on the flight unflustered and safely in tact. If there is a plus for this condition, then this is it. Thanks to the airport authorities for this ingenious service!

One amusing story I recall. At one of the large food stores in London, I was carrying a full basket of groceries on my left arm and unable to carry two wine bottles myself with my right hand. I asked a man in a dark suit to help me, thinking it was one of the staff managers of the department. He was glad to oblige. With charm and good humour, he said he would be 'delighted'. He did so, guided me to the checkout, smiled and left hurriedly. As I was paying, another man came up to me, in a smart dark suit, informing me he was the manager of the food department. 'Madam, do you know who you asked, to carry your wine bottles?' he enquired 'No!' I said, 'why?' He hesitated, and said with a flush of embarrassment, 'That Gentleman is the King of Sweden!' He pointed to a gathering by the cheese counter surrounded by Swedish flags. Red in the face, I awkwardly moved away.

I have since had frequent visits to the hospital as a small wound had developed under my arm, secondary to post-mastectomy radiation. It has been a hindrance and restricted my movements. I had the good fortune to meet two nurses from the hospital, Gwynedd and Anne, who looked after me each time I visited the hospital and attended to and dressed my wound. The care, kindness, common sense and humour overpowered me. One of the most important qualities we need from a nurse is reassurance, coupled with a genuine understanding. With these attributes, Gwynedd and Anne excel.

Subsequently, I had an operation, to remove some mastectomy residual skin which had been causing interference with the mobility of my arm. but this time I was on my own. It was a Saturday morning. I walked to the hospital at 8 a.m. and was prepared for surgery at 9.30 a.m. In this case, during the procedure I was awake and aware. This was a new experience. I had a local anaesthetic. I saw several nurses, surgeons' assistants dressed in their green surgical hats and gowns, moving at speed around me. When the surgeon was attending to my operation, sewing and dressing my wound, I was surprised to hear a buzz, laughter and gossip engaging in conversation of the news of the day. Mubarak was the topic. I was even more surprised to be questioned by the surgeon about my opinion on this subject! I think he was quite vexed I didn't respond!

The operation ended after an hour. I was wheeled into the recovery room and then upstairs and placed on a bed in a regular room. I was given a cup of tea and a sandwich, seen by a staff nurse and told when I had rested and felt strong enough I could go home. At midday I left and started to walk slowly and unsteadily through Marylebone towards home, wanting to adjust to the normality of an ordinary day.

On the way, feeling downcast recalling the morning's ordeal, regardless of it being bright and sunny, a white van drew up and parked by the curb in North Audley Street. A young tall good-looking man hopped out and removed from the back of the van, twenty of the longest-stemmed, salmon-pink roses, with heads so lush and large. From nowhere and for no apparent reason, he simply said, 'These are for you!' Whereupon, he thrust the blooms into my arms. I was speechless. I did manage an incoherent 'thank you' and told him his timing was perfect.

I continued my walk home feeling as though the flawless blooms were a gift from above! After the pain and suffering of the operation that took place earlier, what joy to end the day with warm and loving thoughts of my adored mother!

And now today, as I put pen to paper to end this final chapter, this week I had my check-up at the hospital. A mammogram; an ultra-sound examination; and finally a thorough investigation from my surgeon, Professor Mokbel. There was in existence, a small lump in my existing breast which was in question, but was found unobtrusive. However, the short time I endured waiting for the doctor's comments, I suffered bewilderment and fright which persistently recurred, reflecting the tragic events of the last year. Could I subject myself to all this again? What a question.

If one has to, one does.

Conclusion

My personal journey is coming to an end for the time being.

I asked the experts in the profession to write on their specific subjects, to conclude and refine the canvas of my experience. My gratitude is paramount as without these chapters, there would be no book. It is necessary and important for the reader to have some of their questions answered. Only from the masters would this be possible.

I contacted some of my 'sitters' from my previous publications to express their thoughts, to add a quote, heading the various chapters. I was amazed to find such cooperation from my associates, who have expressed such enthusiasm. I thank them for their words and for giving this book a further dimension.

For myself I have immensely enjoyed writing, bringing together the compilation of authors, and capturing images in order to bring this book to its conclusion.

In order to 'Go with the Flow' we must be brave and – always – optimistic. And as Abraham Lincoln said, 'The best thing about the future is that it comes only one day at a time.'

An Introduction to Gemma Levine's Exercises

JON BOWSKILL BA ACSM FSMT
Specialist in rehabilitation through exercise

As a corrective exercise specialist I work with my team at the Bowskill Clinic to help people from all walks of life, all levels of health, and all levels of activity, from the totally sedentary to the professional athlete. One of the most important parts of what we do with clients is figuring out exactly how to prescribe exercise that will have a beneficial effect on that person's health, well-being or performance.

One of the foundational principles of how we work is based on the premise that the body is designed to move. After all we evolved hunting animals, climbing trees and walking long distances to search for water. The problem is that in modern society we move too little and inefficiently to reap the many benefits that movement can offer.

The human body in itself is an immensely complex system of systems and how we choose to move, or not as the case may be, has a well-established critical effect on our health. Just like many things in life, too much movement can do us just as much harm as too little movement so finding the balance of what is right for each of us as individuals is foundationally important to improving our own health.

When we are sleeping well, have little stress, drink plenty of water, eat a good diet and are free from illness and disease our bodies can cope with quite a lot of exercise and at a relatively high intensity. The less overall stress there is on the human body, the better it can heal, recover and adapt to exercise and therefore respond beneficially. The more stress and strain the body is under, the more difficult it is for the body to recover. Strenuous exercise when your body is under a lot of stress and strain can therefore often have a negative effect on your health, despite the best intentions.

Finding the correct intensity and modality of exercise for your

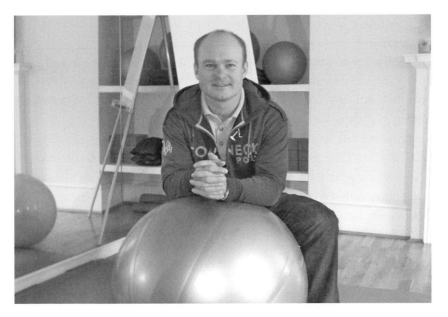

Jon Bowskill

level of well-being then becomes a crucial part of making sure your exercising is making you healthier. As a general rule the more stress and strain your body is under the more gentle and careful you have to be with your exercising.

When you get it right, however, the benefits of correct exercise and movement for those recovering from illness can include:

- Relaxing the nervous system to improve our body's natural healing process
- Reducing stress and anxiety
- Improving the natural flow of lymphatic fluid through the body
- Mobilising and massaging the internal organs through correct breathing technique
- Improving energy and vitality.

When we look to types of exercise that can be beneficial for those recovering from illness it is important that the modality allows maximum opportunity for healing and recovery. Training in water is just one such modality.

Water is very much a part of who we are; we are 80 per cent water at a cellular level, we are born from water and we cannot live without it. For centuries the healing power of water has been used in many forms and there is no doubt that the benefits that it provides are expansive. Stretching and moving in water provides support, comfort and resistance all at the same time. It stimulates the parasympathic branch of the autonomic nervous system responsible for healing and regeneration and allows us to develop flexibility and strength in a supported and gravity-free environment.

Gemma's gentle exercises, which she has evolved from a Swedish technique called *Mensendick*, are examples of how movement within water can be used to help improve strength as well as mobility, cardiovascular health, circulation, relaxation, energy and overall health and well-being.

As with any form of new exercise it is important to get the green light from your doctor first, especially if you have recently been unwell. You should begin the exercises slowly and carefully with close attention to your technique, stopping if you have any adverse symptoms, aches or pains.

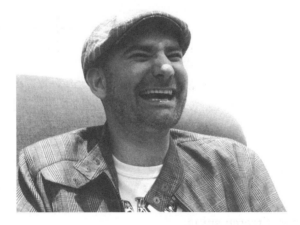

Rikki, who drew the graphics for my exercises

Gemma Levine's Exercises

Pool Exercises

At steps before entering pool.

1 Deep breathing. Sit, straight back, legs apart. Hands on bent knees. Breathe in slowly, hold breath in for count of five. Breathe out slowly and repeat ten times.

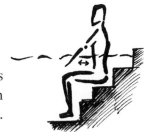

Exercise 1

2 Swim for twenty minutes, favoured style, but be careful not to strain your neck if using breast stroke.

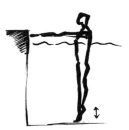

3 Go to side of pool or to a bar at side of pool, water level to be above waist.

Exercise 3a

a) Hold on with both hands and raise feet on to ball of foot and then down, slowly, not quite touching the floor of the pool. Twenty-four times. Exercise foot and calf muscles.

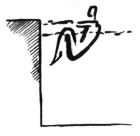

b) Hold on with both hands draw and knees up to chest and down. twenty times. Stretch spine.

Exercise 3b

c) Hold on to bar with right hand and rotate left leg five times and then in opposite direction. Repeat with right leg. Exercise hip joint.

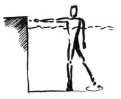

Exercise 3c

d) Hold on to bar with both hands. One knee slightly bent close to bar and other leg stretched out behind with toe (not heel) on base of floor of the pool. Stretch calf muscles to count of twelve. Then other leg.

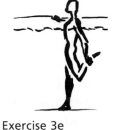

Exercise 3d

e) Hold on to the bar grasp right ankle and pull up and firmly back, drawing the heel towards the buttock. hold to the count of ten. Repeat left leg. Stretch thigh.

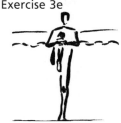

Exercise 3e

f) Lift knee up to chest, as far as possible to stretch back thigh. Hold to count of twelve for each leg.

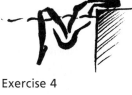

Exercise 3f

4 Find a corner. Place arms outstretched to hold on to both corners (or bar) of the wall of the pool. Follow a, b and c.

Exercise 4

a) Rise up to the top of the water surface on your back. Place both knees together and swing from left to right twenty times, to strengthen obliques.

Exercise 4a

b) Draw legs up to chest then one leg at a time kick with strength forward and back ten times and then the

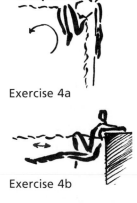

Exercise 4b

other, ten times. Finally both legs together ten times. Kick with as much strength as you can. Good for circulation of lower limbs and strengthening muscles around knee joints.

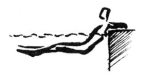

Exercise 4b

c) Draw both legs up and exercise a scissor movement, crossing legs over one another, twenty times. When finished, kick legs vigorously to lower to the floor of the pool. Exercise for the inner thigh

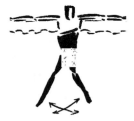

Exercise 4c

5 Go to the deep end and tread water 200 times (a hundred each leg) with elbows and wrists *above* water with hands loosely clenched. This is a difficult exercise and can only be achieved with practice and in time. You might only be able to do five or ten at the beginning. Strengthen stomach muscles.

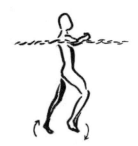

Exercise 5

6 If there are steps: in deep water, hold on to a rail and place your feet on a step at waist level. Push forwards and back-wards, bending knees, twenty times. To strengthen spine and knee joints.

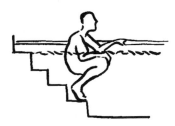

Exercise 6

7a) Standing with water above waist level, rotate one shoulder five times, then in the opposite direction. Repeat, the other shoulder. Strengthen shoulder muscles.

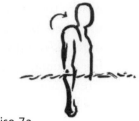

Exercise 7a

7b) Rotate head five times to the right, then to the left. Exercise neck.

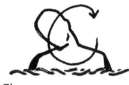

Exercise 7b

7c) With both arms at the same time, clench fists, rotate arms 'out' and then 'in'. Eight times. Rotate both wrists left and right five times each way. Then hold your hands as if praying, push gently down to the left and then the right. Eight times. Then the same with the thumbs, pressing the top inner soft part of the thumb hard against each other, eight times. Finish by shaking wrists vigorously.

    Finish this exercise, by tightly gripping your hands behind your back and pulling in your shoulder blades firmly. Elbows nearly touching. Exercise chest muscles. Release and repeat ten times.

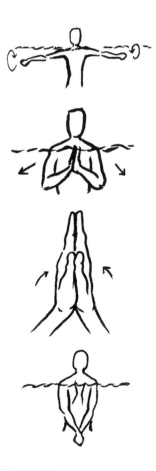

Exercise 7c

8 Finally, return to the steps.

a) Lift one leg first, on to a step higher than the waist and with a straight leg, push down at the knee eight times, then the other leg. Strengthen back calf and knees.

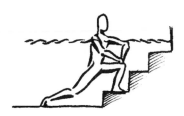

Exercise 8a

b) On step 3, crouch (squat) with knees bent and rise up and down in a bobbing movement, 30 times. Strengthen thighs, ham strings and knees.

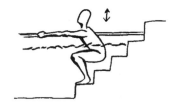

Exercise 8b

c) Sit on step and clench your buttock muscles tightly and then release ten times.

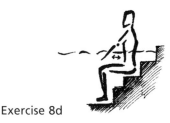

Exercise 8c

d) Repeat deep breathing exercises same as, No. 1 at the start of the course. Will enable you to relax before leaving.

Exercise 8d

SMILE!

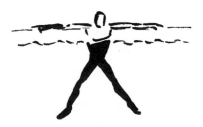

Special Exercises for Post Mastectomy

These exercises should take fifteen minutes. '*An extra one for luck*' – I always count an extra one . . . one to ten and an extra one for luck!

These exercises (also in the pool) for a further ten minutes, can be added on to the previous exercises. It will be good to use side stroke and breast stroke in moderation for post mastectomy. Exclude the crawl.

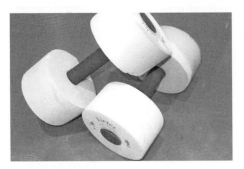

Water resistance weights

1 Take 'foam ball' resistance weights.
2 One in each hand, alternatively, draw up and down, side of thigh and leg. ten times.
3 One in each hand, draw arms out and back towards shoulder blades, then pull both foam weights to meet in centre front of the body. ten times to start, then add as the weeks go by.
4 One foam ball weight in each hand, alternative arm movements, stretch forward and back just skimming under the water surface. This exercise is stronger than the former ones, and 'can' be excluded at the start, but try five and then build up through the weeks.

These exercises outside the pool. No ball weights needed.

5 Find a pillar or wall, stand upright. With your hands and arms,

with fingers 'creepy crawly' movements, climb the wall, as high as you can. When you reach a required height, hold for five seconds and then back, down the wall, twenty times.

6   Clasp both hands together above your head and slowly swing to the left then right. Ten times.

7   Clasp your hands together, behind you at buttocks level, and gently flex your elbows to meet one another. Ten times.

8   Interlock your hands behind your neck and stretch your elbows out to the side. Bring elbows back into the centre. Five times. This is a strong exercise.

These exercises should, after some months, relieve the tightness of your skin (where the stitches were) to enable your body to feel less tense and your skin more supple. It is important that you start slowly and as the weeks go by, as you get stronger, gradually build up on the counts. Always, one extra for luck!

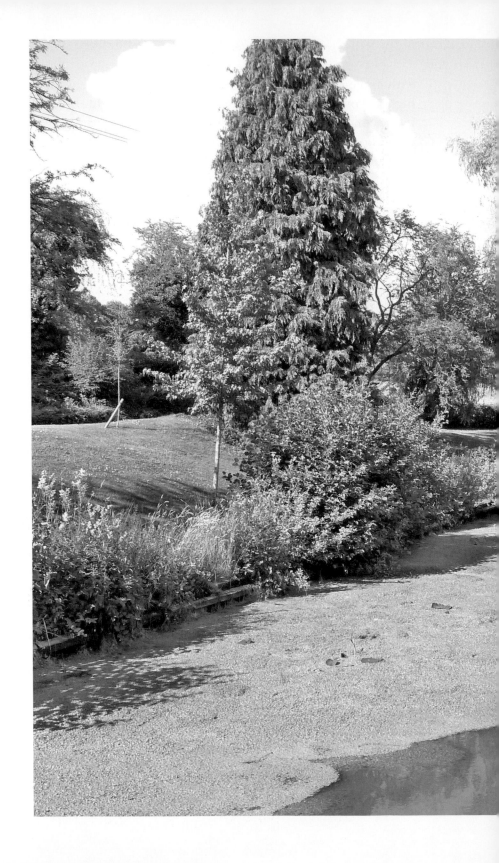

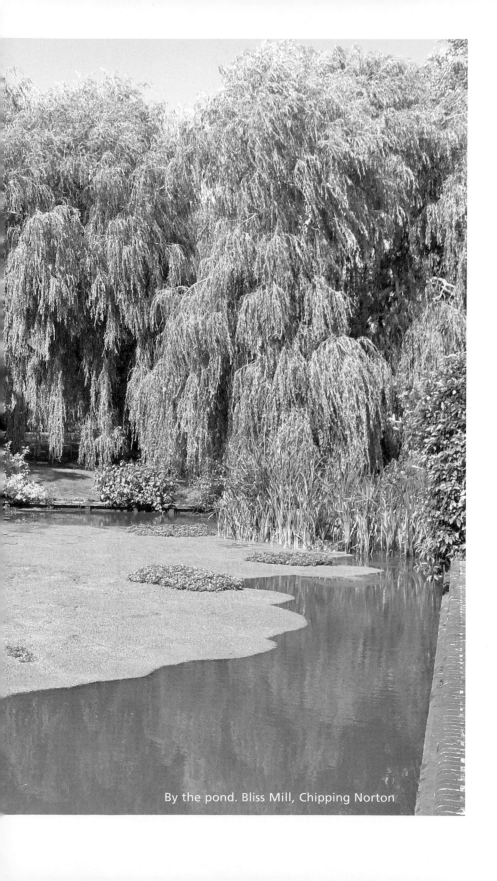

By the pond. Bliss Mill, Chipping Norton

Envoi

Mum: 1 Cancer: 0

JAMES

For all I've seen and all I've known,
Of all the ills and sadness shown,
To see once more the garden grown,
What better, what more, what else to ask for?

ADAM